Glaxo Pharmaceuticals™
DIVISION OF GLAXO INC

Five Moore Drive, P.O. Box 13438
Research Triangle Park, NC 27709
Telex 802813
Phone (919) 248-2100
Fax (919) 248-2381

J. Stanley Hull
Director of Marketing
Gastrointestinal Products

Dear Doctor:

Glaxo is pleased to sponsor the publication of the text
Gastrointestinal Endoscopy by John Baillie, M.B., Ch.B., F.R.C.P.
(Glasg.). In addition to our pharmaceutical products, we are
committed to providing support for continuing medical education
in the field of gastroenterology.

Dr. Baillie has done an excellent job in writing this book and we
are sure the information will provide an excellent overview of
endoscopic procedures and techniques.

We wish you every success in your future in the field of
gastroenterology.

Sincerely,

J. Stanley Hull
Director of Marketing
Gastrointestinal Products
Glaxo Pharmaceuticals

Gastrointestinal Endoscopy
Basic principles and practice

Presented
with the Compliments of

Glaxo

To _____

By _____

For Alison

Gastrointestinal Endoscopy

Basic principles and practice

John Baillie BSc(Hons), MB, ChB, FRCP(Glasg.)

Associate Director of Gastrointestinal Endoscopy,
Division of Gastroenterology, Duke University Medical Center,
Durham, North Carolina, USA

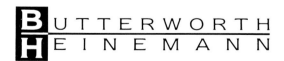

Butterworth-Heinemann Ltd
Linacre House, Jordan Hill, Oxford OX2 8DP

 PART OF REED INTERNATIONAL BOOKS

OXFORD   LONDON   BOSTON
MUNICH   NEW DELHI   SINGAPORE   SYDNEY
TOKYO   TORONTO   WELLINGTON

First published 1992

British Library Cataloguing in Publication Data
Baillie, John
  Gastrointestinal Endoscopy: Basic
  Principles and Practice
  I. Title
  616.07

ISBN 0 7506 1357 2

Library of Congress Cataloging in Publication
Baillie, John
  Gastrointestinal endoscopy: basic principles and practice/by
  John Baillie.
  p.   cm.
  Includes bibliographical references and index.
  ISBN 0 7506 1357 2
  1. Endoscopy.   2. Gastrointestinal system – Diseases – Diagnosis.
  I. Title.
  [DNLM: 1. Endoscopy, Gastrointestinal – methods.
  2. Gastrointestinal Diseases – diagnosis.   WI 141 B157q]
  RC804.E6B35
  616.3'307545–dc20
  DNLM/DLC
  for Library of Congress   92–8067
                                                                  CIP

Printed and bound in Great Britain by The Bath Press, Avon

Contents

Foreword

The trainee physician's introduction to gastrointestinal endoscopic procedures can be both a frustrating and intimidating experience. Today's
sophisticated GI endoscopy laboratory contains an awesome array of
instrumentation, endoscopic paraphernalia, and well-trained support personnel. In any uncharted and unexplored territory, an accurate map and
concise 'trip-ticket' are invaluable. It was with this goal in mind that John
Baillie developed this book, *Gastrointestinal Endoscopy: Basic Principles
and Practice*.

Dr Baillie's background in endoscopic teaching and computer simulated
modeling spans two continents and encompasses a rich and varied endoscopic training experience. Recognizing the trials and tribulations common to
the endoscopic tyro, he felt compelled to develop an endoscopic manual
which accurately charts a course through the learning phase of endoscopy
and beyond. The performance of an endoscopic procedure requires
manual dexterity and hand–eye coordination. The clinical relevance of an
endoscopic procedure relies upon the visual prowess, interpretive skills
and attention to detail of the physician operator. The art of endoscopy is a
combination of both of these elements. In his endoscopy manual, Dr
Baillie has incorporated many of these elements which he and others have
perfected through their endoscopic learning experience. He first intro-
duces the 'tools of the trade' to the beginner. He then develops a
step-by-step approach to performing the specific endoscopic procedure
including the necessary maneuvering and interpretive assessment of the
endoscopic anatomy and pathology.

John Baillie has written this manual in a simply designed, very readable
and easily understood format for the beginner to endoscopy. This endoscopic manual is a most useful tool for introducing gastrointestinal endoscopy
to the student physician. Although there are enough unique observations
and 'tricks of the trade' included in this manual to interest the 'so-called'
expert in gastrointestinal endoscopy, Dr Baillie's main focus is to present
the initial experience in gastrointestinal endoscopy in a crisp, practical
manner. He has long wished to set his many talents in endoscopic teaching
to paper. I think this book has adequately accomplished this goal.

Walter J. Hogan MD
Professor of Medicine
Division of Gastroenterology
Medical College of Wisconsin
USA

Preface

The evolution of gastrointestinal (GI) endoscopy since the introduction of flexible fiberoptic endoscopes 30 years ago has been spectacular. What started as a purely diagnostic technique has blossomed into a highly complex subspecialty within gastroenterology. Although we must be first and foremost well-trained clinicians, the ever-increasing sophistication of GI endoscopy dictates the need for broad-based training and experience.

This basic textbook of GI endoscopy is written by a teacher of endoscopy with the trainee in mind. However, I hope that it may provide established endoscopists with food for thought as well. It is not intended to be encyclopedic, nor is it yet another atlas of endoscopic photographs. Instead, I have tried to address the frequent complaint of endoscopic trainees that standard textbooks often ignore the 'tricks of the trade'. There is certainly no substitute for 'hands on' experience, nor for the input of expert teachers of endoscopy in the learning process. However, if this book succeeds in filling in just a few of the gaps encountered in even the best training programs, it will have achieved its goal. The astute will notice conspicuous omissions: endoscopic ultrasound does not feature, and many of the more sophsiticated therapeutic procedures (e.g. laser photocoagulation, pancreatic duct stenting) are mentioned only in passing. This is intentional. These are advanced procedures requiring additional (third tier) training.

The bibliography provided at the end of each chapter is a starting point only: the voracious reader will find exhaustive literature reviews in the larger textbooks of endoscopy. To limit the text to a manageable size, I chose not to duplicate information easily accessible elsewhere, e.g. the physics of electrocautery, lists of equipment makers and suppliers and the names and addresses of professional organizations.

The American Society of Gastrointestinal Endoscopy (ASGE) has played a major role in addressing the many difficult issues related to training and certification of endoscopists. As a committed teacher of endoscopy, I applaud the pursuit of excellence represented by ASGE training guidelines. The text of this book was extensively rewritten to incorporate emerging ASGE recommendations. I thank the President and Governing Board of the ASGE for permission to reproduce and abstract these guidelines, which I regard as the foundation for a renaissance in endoscopic training. Students of endoscopy are encouraged to use this book to familiarize themselves with the basics. For greater detail, a variety of excellent textbooks and atlases are available. It is my hope that teachers of endoscopy will find this book helpful and an accessible source of information for their trainees.

In particular, I wish to recognize the superb teaching skills of Kenneth Cochran, Roger Gebhard, Robert Mackie, Jim Pries, Jack Vennes, Steve Silvis. In addition, I have been blessed with many fine mentors and friends, notably David Fleischer, Joe Geenen, Jerry Waye, Christopher Williams, Willie Webb, Kees Huibregtse and Guido Tytgat. Outstanding GI nurses have greatly influenced my practice: in particular, Lois Nelson, Nancy Shields, Mary Bond and Marsha Dreyer smoothed off many rough edges during my Fellowship training. I wish to thank Pat Minchin (Edgware Hospital, London) for many helpful ideas and comments and Pat Mitchel (The Middlesex Hospital, London) for sharing her extensive knowledge of ERCP equipment and accessories.

My former teacher and now colleague at Duke, Dr Peter Cotton, has been a staunch supporter from the beginning; for his friendship, example and good humor, I thank him sincerely. I am also deeply indebted to an old friend and mentor, Dr Walter Hogan, Past President of the ASGE, who reviewed the first draft of the book and made many valuable suggestions. In particular, the sections detailing the endoscopic anatomy of the pharynx, esophagus and stomach greatly benefitted from his input. I thank Dr Ian Taylor, MD, PhD, Chief of the Division of Gastroenterology at Duke for supporting my academic activities, including the completion of this book. A good friend, an inspired teacher and the busiest man I know, Dick Kozarek of Seattle, generously found time to review this manuscript and provide insightful comments.

It has been my privilege to teach many fine young physicians passing through the GI Fellowship program at Duke. They taught me much along the way. I have to thank two of the best, Drs John Affronti and Stan Branch, for reviewing the manuscript and providing many helpful suggestions.

Just as 'no man is an island', no author can flourish without an inspired editor: I cannot overestimate the contribution of Dr Geoffrey Smaldon, PhD, a man with infinite patience and optimism. I am most grateful to Michael Maddalena and Chris Jarvis of Butterworth-Heinemann for their expertise and attention to detail. The excellent line drawings that accompany the text bear testimony to the skill of Ms Stacy Kerr and the publishers and I gratefully acknowledge the assistance of Glaxo Pharmaceuticals in the funding of the illustrations. The financial support of Glaxo Pharmaceuticals will render this textbook widely available to trainees in endoscopy. The manuscript, which required seemingly endless revision, would probably have foundered without the tireless efforts of my wonderful secretary, Ms Lynn Foster. Finally, I must thank my wife, Alison, for her support and encouragement, and apologize to my children, Katie and Christopher, who saw little of their father while this book was being written.

This book is divided into four chapters: Chapter 1 discusses issues common to all endoscopic procedures. Chapters 2, 3 and 4 cover Upper GI Endoscopy, Colonoscopy and Endoscopic Retrograde Cholangiopancreatography (ERCP), respectively. As the emphasis is on basics, I have tried to limit the discussion of therapeutic procedures. However, making a distinction between purely diagnostic procedures and those involving some therapy is rather artificial. In the late 1960s and early 1970s, GI endoscopy evolved from a largely diagnostic field into one with a major therapeutic role. Therapeutic endoscopy provides a safe and effective alternative to surgery in many circumstances. The spectrum of therapeutic endoscopy ranges from dilatation of benign esophageal strictures and decompression of colonic pseudo-obstruction to palliation of malignant biliary obstruction and laser ablation of gut tumors. Many of these procedures require advanced training; the discussion of therapy has been directed towards the most commonly used techniques. Inevitably the style and content of any textbook reflects the interests and prejudices of the author; this book is no exception.

1

Introduction

Endoscopes and accessories

Flexible endoscopes have become very sophisticated but retain a basic design that has proved effective over the years (Figure 1.1). A recent major innovation has been the introduction of video imaging as an alternative to fiberoptics. Endoscopes have a control head which includes an eyepiece (in fiberoptic instruments only), and wheels and buttons to control tip movement and air/water and suction respectively. Lateral viewing endoscopes have an elevator. The control head is connected to a flexible shaft with a maneuverable tip. A connecting (umbilical) cord provides illumination from a static light source, as well as air, water and suction.

In video endoscopes, the eypiece is redundant; the endoscope is held at waist level and the image is viewed on a television monitor (Figure 1.2). In place of the eyepiece, there are a variety of buttons that control video recording and other image management systems (Figure 1.3). To be effective, endoscopes require the right combination of thickness, proximal stiffness and distal flexibility. For example, most endoscopes used for upper GI tract work (e.g. gastroscopes, duodenoscopes) have an external diameter in the range of 8–11 mm. Thinner endoscopes are available for pediatric work and to access strictures, but their small diameter has drawbacks. Pediatric endoscopes suffer from excessive flexibility, reduced

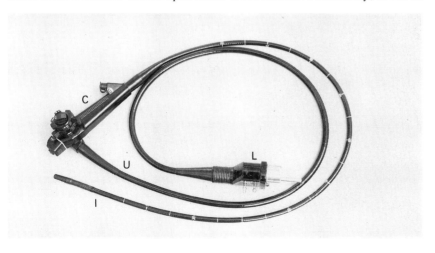

Figure 1.1 Endoscope design. C, control head (in this instance a video endoscope); U, umbilical cord; L, light source attachment; I, insertion tube

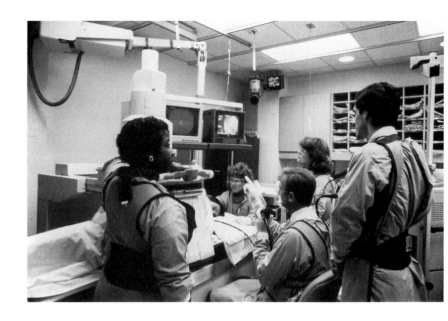

Figure 1.2 The benefits of video endoscopy. Everyone involved can watch the procedure. Note the convenient side-by-side arrangement of the X-ray and video monitors

image quality, a small instrument channel (limiting biopsy size), and tend to be damaged more easily than standard 'adult' instruments. Colono-scopes have different requirements. Again, contrary to expectations, flexibility is a mixed blessing. To prevent looping and to straighten out existing bends in the colon, the proximal part of the insertion tube should be quite stiff. As the lumen of the colon is significantly larger than that of the esophagus or duodenum, the external diameter of a colonoscope can be proportionately larger (e.g. 15 mm). Pediatric colonoscopes (e.g. 10 mm external diameter) can prove invaluable when tight strictures limit access with a standard instrument, but they have significant limitations in routine use. Colonoscopes also come in a variety of sizes, ranging from the

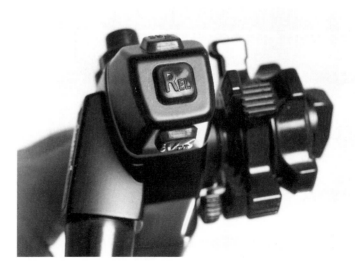

Figure 1.3 Control head of video endoscope

'long' (165–180 cm) to the 'short' (70–110 cm). The latter is used almost exclusively for flexible sigmoidoscopy. Medium and long instruments are required for full colonoscopy; which type is used is a matter of personal preference, the long variety being somewhat stiffer. All endoscopes have an instrument channel with an opening in the control head (Figure 1.4). The standard channel diameter is around 2–3 mm, although endoscopes used for therapeutic procedures have large instrument channels of 3.7 mm diameter or greater. Endoscopes with two instrument channels are available for specialized procedures such as difficult polypectomy (requiring two snares) and management of acute GI bleeding. The instrument channel is easily blocked by solid matter, including food debris and blood clot. If flushing with water (using a standard syringe with a long tip) does not clear a blockage, the problem is usually in the umbilical cord. To unblock this, the system needs to be flushed from the air/water connector at the light source end. Expensive maintenance 'down time' can be avoided by rigorous cleaning and air drying of endoscopes between procedures, which prevents accumulation of dried debris.

Side-viewing endoscopes used for duodenoscopy have a small elevator (or bridge) at the distal end of the instrument channel that allows the operator some movement of devices (e.g. biopsy forceps, papillotomes)

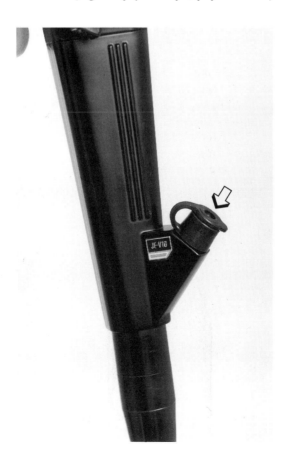

Figure 1.4 Instrument port (arrowed)

advanced down the endoscope. This bridge is independently controlled by a lever on the control head, adjacent to the control wheels (Figure 1.5).

Illumination is provided by a unit that combines a light source (either xenon arc or halogen–tungsten) with an air and water pump (Figure 1.6). These units allow the intensity of illumination to be varied, as well as the force of air insufflation.

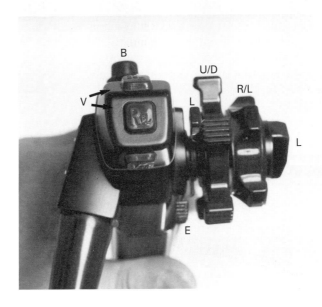

Figure 1.5 Instrument control head from above. V, video management control buttons; B, suction button (air/water button below this – hidden); E, elevator control level; U/D, up–down control wheel; R/L, right–left control wheel; L, control wheel lock

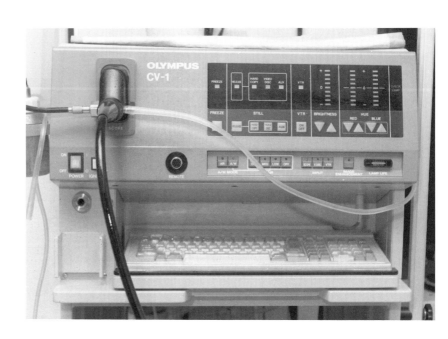

Figure 1.6 Video endoscope light source (Olympus CV-1)

Accessories

There are multiple accessories available to the endoscopist, including biopsy forceps, cytology brushes, snares, balloons, baskets, sclerotherapy needles, etc. The size of these devices is limited by the diameter of the endoscope instrument channel. Endoscopic biopsy forceps (Figure 1.7) comprise sharpened cups connected to a central handle by a metal cable. The size of the biopsy is limited by the length of the cups which have to be able to pass through the instrument channel. A cytology brush is basically a plastic sleeve through which the brush is advanced and into which it can be retracted for removal (Figure 1.8). Endoscopic accessories required for specific procedures will be described in the relevant sections.

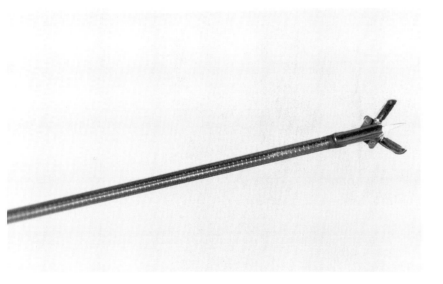

Figure 1.7 Biopsy forceps with central 'prong'

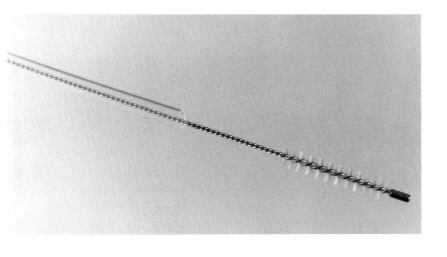

Figure 1.8 Endoscopic cytology brush

Holding an endoscope

The standard 'grip' or position for holding the endoscope is illustrated in Figure 1.9. The control piece is placed in the left hand with the fourth and fifth fingers lightly holding the instrument. This leaves the index (second) and middle finger free to activate the air/water and suction buttons, respectively. The control wheels can be moved with the thumb and index finger, leaving the right hand free to hold the insertion tube. In practice, the right hand is used from time to time for control wheel inputs. However, the beginner should get comfortable with the grip and be able to adjust the control wheels mainly with the right hand. Endoscope design allows the transmission of torque (twist) from the control head to the tip. The

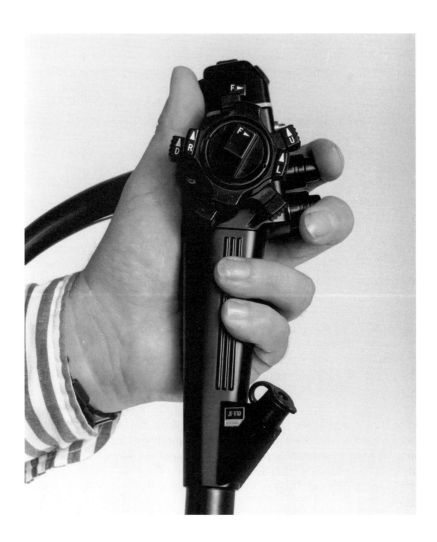

Figure 1.9 'The grip'. Index and middle fingers left free to activate suction and air/water buttons, respectively

application of torque both from the control head (by wrist action) and the insertion tube greatly increase the versatility of the instrument. The field of view of an endoscope depends on the nature of the lens at the tip. This is usually a wide angle lens (90–130°) which focuses the endoscopic image on to the fiber bundle. The depth of field varies from a few millimeters to around 15 cm. A focussing lens system in the eyepiece of a fiberoptic endoscope allows the image to be adjusted for individual users. There is no focus adjustment on video endoscopes. It is important to avoid getting lubricating gel on the lens surface, as this may distort the image.

Fiberoptics versus video imaging

Until recently, all flexible endoscopes employed fiberoptic bundles both for illumination and image transmission. A fiberoptic bundle contains in excess of 20 000 plastic-coated glass fibers of approximately 10 μm diameter. These fibers are coated with opaque material to prevent loss of light by refraction through the surface. As long as the orientation of the fibers in the bundle remains the same (collimated), an image can be transmitted through the bundle, regardless of twists and turns.

There are intrinsic drawbacks of fiberoptics, including image resolution limited by the size and number of fibers, fragility, loss of light transmission properties with age and X-ray exposure, suceptibility to contamination with water and, of course, the dependence of an eyepiece. Video endoscope imaging employs light sensitive electronic 'chips', or charge coupled devices (CCDs) on the tip of the endoscope. Collectively, many thousands of light sensitive points (pixels) create high resolution television images. Early video endoscopes used a cumbersome system with rapid, sequential image filtering to create a pseudo-color image. Unfortunately, this tended to create an unpleasant stroboscopic effect under certain conditions. So-called color CCD chips have overcome this problem; these chips are modified with colored filters that render individual pixels sensitive to only one of the three primary colors (red, green and blue). A true color television image can now be created without flicker effect. The image resolution and clarity of video endoscopes is impressive, and can only improve with refinements in technology. Video endoscopes are more comfortable to use than fiberoptic ones and allow assistants and trainees to watch procedures on a television monitor instead of through a cumbersome teaching attachment. Video endoscope illumination is still provided by fiberoptics, but the days of fiberoptic imaging are numbered. However, until the transition to video technology is complete, fiberoptic instruments can be used with video monitors by attaching a television convertor to the eyepiece (Figure 1.10). Modern endoscopy units have an array of audio-visual aids to complement this dazzling imagery, including devices to make 'hard copy' of 'frozen' images (e.g. Mavigraph[TM]) and video tapes of interesting cases.

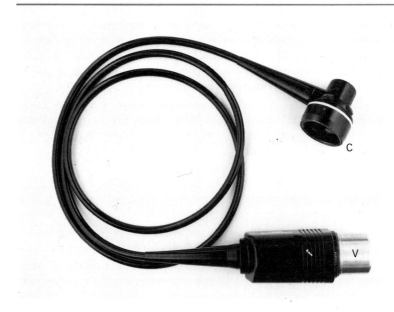

Figure 1.10 Video convertor. C, eyepiece convertor attachment; V, video processor input

Endoscopy unit design and function

There has been growing interest in the design and function of GI endoscopy units. This reflects the need for careful planning to insure efficient and effective flow. Provision has to be made not only for performing endoscopic procedures themselves, but also for pre- and postprocedure management of patients and those accompanying them. The facilities required include (but are not limited to) a reception and waiting area, space for patients to undress and be assessed before each procedure, endoscopy rooms (some equipped with fluoroscopy), a supervised recovery area, interview rooms for predischarge discussion, a reporting area (for generating procedure reports) and (by no means least) changing, toilet, rest and office facilities for endoscopy unit staff. With the increasing sophistication of endoscopic procedures, many units have a patient education area, where video tapes can be viewed and written materials reviewed. As the amount of information generated by a modern endoscopy unit is formidable, provision must be made for data management. Increasingly, patient data is being kept in computer memory. Although even small desk-top microcomputers can store a large volume of data, a busy endoscopy unit can quickly fill available hard disc memory. In the near future optical storage media will replace the computer hard disc, as these have enormous memory capability (e.g. one compact disc (CD) can store the equivalent of 550 Megabytes of data).

Endoscopy units require an organized way of handling audiovisual materials. With the advent of the video endoscopy era, endoscopic images which used to be captured on 35 mm color slides are now being printed as ard copy (e.g. Mavigraph) or recorded on video tape. In addition, both endoscopic and fluoroscopic images can now be stored in digital form. Without an organized system to document and store this mass of audio-visual material, chaos quickly ensues! Image management systems are one (expensive) solution. Where the volume and diversity of materials justify it, the appointment of a staff member to oversee audiovisual activities is highly recommended.

How do we judge the effectiveness of an endoscopy unit? This cannot simply be a function of the volume of cases alone, or the income generated from procedures. Sivak has offered the concept of the 'procedure unit', which describes every activity involved in patient management from booking procedures to mailing out reports to referring physicians. Any estimate of the cost effectiveness of an endoscopy unit must take into account the activities of all unit personnel, including desk clerks, secretaries, nurses, GI assistants, physicians, etc. The financial health and efficiency of any endoscopy unit depends on a highly complex equation.

Quality assurance (QA) is a major issue in the 1990s, and is a very important reason for keeping accurate, up-to-date records. QA monitors patient safety, physician competence and the appropriateness of the procedures we perform. Many physicians are suspicious of QA because they feel that 'big brother' is watching them. However, QA merely formalizes what good physicians have been doing for years: continuously assessing their performance against established standards and learning from experience of adverse outcomes.

Finally, the educational activities of the endoscopy unit should not be forgotten. At one end of the spectrum, large academic units often run courses for trainee and established endoscopists to demonstrate the latest techniques, usually with advanced audiovisual aids. However, even the smallest endoscopy unit can (and should) have an active educational program for its own staff and interested local physicians; regular reviews of interesting cases and evolving techniques, with the occasional lecture by a visiting expert, serve to maintain interest and expertise.

Conscious sedation

The success of the many simple and complex procedures currently performed by endoscopists depends on the use of conscious sedation, i.e. the administration of drugs that allow the introduction and manipulation of endoscopes yet provide a relaxed patient, able to respond and maintain vital functions. To address the many practical issues involved in conscious sedation, the ASGE developed the following guidelines in 1989:

1 A well-trained gastrointestinal assistant, working closely with the physician, who observes the patient's status during endoscopic procedures, is the most important part of the monitoring process.
2 The use of extracorporeal equipment to monitor patients may be a useful adjunct to patient surveillance, but is never a substitute for clinical assessment.

3 The amount of monitoring should be proportional to the perceived risk to the individual patient undergoing each specific procedure.
4 The minimal clinical monitoring for all sedated patients should include heart rate, blood pressure and respiratory rate.
5 The proper role for pulse oximetry and continuous electrocardiogram (EKG) monitoring is controversial. Given the cost of the equipment and the manpower to use it, the best decision as to whether it should be used would be based on data exhibiting that such monitoring affects patient outcomes. Such data do not exist
6 However, in those situations in which the individualized need of the patient indicates that more frequent assessment of cardiac rhythm or oxygen saturation will complement the clinical assessment, use of EKG monitoring or pulse oximetry may be beneficial.

The pulse oximeter is an electronic monitoring device now widely used in endoscopy units. A probe clipped on to one of the patient's fingers measures capillary oxygen saturation and pulse rate. These values are continuously updated and displayed prominently on the front of a monitor. During prolonged endoscopic procedures, which are usually performed in a darkened room, pulse oximetry often provides the first indication of oxygen desaturation and changes in pulse rate. Persistent tachycardia is one indication of patient discomfort. Although it has yet to be shown that pulse oximetry alters patient outcome related to endoscopy, it is reassuring to the endoscopist and assistants to have this information. Intermittent automated blood pressure (BP) and continuous EKG monitoring are available in some units. Although pre- and postprocedure BP measurements are standard, it has not been demonstrated that routine monitoring of BP during endoscopy affects outcome. Similarly, with the exception of patients with specific cardiac risk factors, routine EKG monitoring is probably unnecessary.

Drugs used for conscious sedation

The choice of drug or drugs you use for conscious sedation is less important than familiarity with them. Endoscopists must know the pharmacology, indications and contraindications, recommended dosage, duration of action, known side-effects and methods of reversal (if available) for each drug they use. Most endoscopists have their 'favorite' drugs, with which they and their assistants become familiar. When a new sedative agent is introduced, great care must be taken to avoid problems. In particular, those administering the new drug must adhere strictly to the recommended dosage and rate of infusion. As a hypothetical example of the danger of a cavalier approach, an assistant who does not appreciate that the new drug needs to be titrated slowly to achieve a desired response may give a bolus dose, resulting in apnea. Table 1.1 provides a list of drugs commonly used for conscious sedation. (Note that this table is provided for comparison and general information, and should *not* be used for patient management.) Drugs used to control secretions and motility have not been included in this list. For many years, atropine was used routinely as premedication for

Table 1.1 Comparison of sedative agents used for conscious sedation

Drug	Type	Dose	Reverse with naloxone?	Adverse reaction
Meperidine (Demerol)	Narcotic	0.5–1.0 mg/kg i.v. over 2–3 minutes then repeat q. 30 minutes	YES	Respiratory depression, tachycardia, GI upset
Diazepam (Valium)	Benzodiazepine	1–10 mg i.v. slowly over 5 minutes; may repeat q. 30 minutes†	NO	Respiratory depression, hypotension, decreased tolerance in elderly
Midazolam (Versed)	Benzodiazepine	0.5–1.0 mg i.v. over 2–3 minutes, then titrate small doses*	NO	Apnea, confusion, diminished reflexes
Promethazine (Phenergan)	Antihistamine	12.5–25 mg i.v. over 1 minute†	NO	Somnolence, confusion, nausea, potentiates CNS depressants
Diphen-ydramine (Benadryl)	Antihistamine	25–50 mg i.v. over 1 minute†	NO	As above
Fentanyl (Sublimaze)	Opiod analgesic	20–50 μg i.v. over 1–2 minutes, then repeat q. 30 minutes	YES	Respiratory depression, bradycardia, nausea
Droperidol (Inapsine)	Neuroleptic tranquilizer	1.25–2.5 mg i.v. over 1–2 minutes, then repeat q. 30 minutes	NO	Hypotension, tachycardia, restlessness, extra-pyramidal signs

This table is provided for comparison and general information, but should *not* be used for patient management. Physicians must check specific dosage and administration guidelines (package insert) for each drug prior to clinical use.

The elderly and patients with chronic respiratory disease are especially sensitive to benzodiazepines; as little as 1 mg of diazepam given i.v. may cause respiratory depression.
Dose of antihistamines should be reduced for patients over 60 years of age.

ndoscopy. However, a long duration of action and unpleasant side-effects (dry mouth, visual and bladder disturbance) made it unpopular with patients. A hyoscine derivative with shorter action and few side-effects, Buscopan (hyoscine *N*-butylbromide), has been available for over a decade in Europe but sadly has never been approved for use in the USA. A slow intravenous injection of 0.5–1.0 mg of glucagon provides brief but useful control of gut motility. As glucagon is short acting, this can be repeated several times during a prolonged procedure. Finally, many physicians like to use pharyngeal anesthesia in the form of a lozenge, spray or viscous solution to inhibit the gag reflex for upper GI endoscopy (esophagogastro duodenoscopy, EGD). Despite flavoring, most of these lidocaine (lignocaine)-based agents have a bitter after-taste. Their duration of useful action is approximately 30–90 minutes. Patients must be advised not to eat or drink until the effect of pharyngeal sedation has completely worn off.

Recovery

Supervising recovery from procedures performed under conscious sedation is an important function of the endoscopy nurse or assistant. Most modern endoscopy units have a recovery area where patients can be monitored by designated individual. Outpatients must be monitored until they are sufficiently alert and mobile to leave with an escort. After an initial period of immediate postprocedure supervision, hospital inpatients can be sent back to their rooms to complete their recovery. However, this should only be done if arrangements can be made to provide a similar standard of supervision until complete recovery. Patients should not be returned to their hospital room to recover if a nurse cannot be provided to monitor their progress; the ward must provide a similar level of supervision to that available in the endoscopy unit.

It is helpful to provide outpatients with an information sheet when they leave the endoscopy unit. Patients and their family members often fail to assimilate postprocedure instructions, and recently sedated patients may have little or no recollection of discussing the procedure and its outcome with their physician before leaving. The information sheet can provide details of the procedure as well as standard postprocedure instructions (e.g. about diet, activity), follow-up appointments and instructions in the event of problems developing later. It is particularly useful to provide the name and telephone (or pager) number of the physician responsible for dealing with out-of-hours emergencies.

ASGE endoscopic training guidelines

Statement of endoscopic training

The objective of endoscopic training programs is to provide critical supervised instruction in GI endoscopy. Endoscopic procedures are not isolated technical activities, but must be regarded by instructor and trainee as integral aspects of clinical problem-solving. Endoscopic decision-making and technical proficiency are equally important, and the interdependence of these skills must be emphasized repeatedly during the training period.

The basic requirements for successful programs are: (1) skilled, experienced, endoscopic supervisors who continually maintain and improve their abilities; (2) trainees with sound general medical or surgical training who have the motivation and aptitutude for endoscopy; (3) a structured training experience with ongoing evaluation of each trainee's progress in relation to interests, aptitudes and career goals; and (4) opportunity for adequate clinical experience. Not all programs need to provide training in all endoscopic procedures to each trainee.

Important features of a training program

Training personnel

The endoscopy training supervisor should be a sound clinician and teacher who is well trained, experienced and skilled in endoscopy. The supervisor should be responsible for: (a) appropriate didactic instruction; (b) supervision of all elective and emergency cases; (c) continued instruction in endoscopic decision-making, technique and interpretation of findings; and (d) ongoing evaluation of procedures, reports and photographic records. The supervisor's judgement will determine when the trainee may progress from directly supervised to less closely supervised and, finally, to independent procedures. Upon completion of training, the supervisor will determine if the trainee is qualified to perform independent GI endoscopy.

Additional endoscopic instructions should be available, when needed, to provide general supervision or specific expertise.

A gastrointestinal assistant should be available to assist with procedures and to aid in instruction regarding maintenance of endoscopic equipment.

Endoscopic training should take place within the framework of clinical care and problem solving

Endoscopic procedures should be preceded by a careful clinical evaluation, including indications and individual risk factors; most often this should be carried out by the trainee and reviewed by the supervisor.

Indications, contraindications and benefit–risk considerations should be reviewed with a supervisor before each endoscopy.

Sensitivity to cost–benefit considerations and appropriate sequencing of endoscopic and other procedures are important elements in diagnostic and therapeutic decision-making that should be emphasized throughout the period of training. Deciding when *not* to perform endoscopy is an important aspect of endoscopic training.

The trainee should learn to explain the endoscopic procedure to the patient, including the obtaining of informed consent.

The trainee should carry out the immediate postendoscopy evaluation of the patient, and the program should provide for follow-up evaluation wherever possible.

Endoscopic findings should be discussed with the physician responsible for the patient's care.

Technical proficiency must be acquired in a sequential fashion.

1 Trainees should receive instruction in (a) endoscopic anatomy, (b) technic
  features and capabilities of endoscopic equipment, and (c) accessory endoscop
  techniques including biopsy, cytology, photography and electrosurgery.
2 Trainees should observe endoscopic procedures before performing them. In
  struction in premedication, preparation of the patient, close monitoring o
  sedated patients, and the effects of endoscopy on coexisting medical problems
  essential at this stage of training.
3 Trainees should perform each type of endoscopic procedure under dire
  supervision before performing them independently.
4 Systematic correlation of endoscopic findings with radiographic and patholog
  data (surgical specimens, biopsy and cytology material) should be part of eac
  endoscopy.
5 The trainee shall participate in the preparation of complete written repor
  immediately following each endoscopic procedure.
6 Photographic documentation of lesions should be part of endoscopic procedure
  and reviewed with the supervisor.

Endoscopic facility

An endoscopic facility should be available as described in the ASG
Guidelines for Establishment of Gastrointestinal Endoscopy Areas.

Additional requirements

1 Records of all procedures, findings and complications should be maintained.
2 Regular conferences should provide for critical discussion of endoscopic case
  complications and deaths.
3 Teaching collections should be developed, including clinical summaries, endo
  scopic photographs and relevant radiographic and pathologic material.
4 Records of each trainee's performance should be maintained and reviewed wit
  the trainee periodically.
5 Endoscopic research strengthens the training experience and should be include
  in the program.

Statement on the role of short courses in endoscopic training

A short course is defined as an organized training program lasting less tha
several weeks, and often only a few days.

The rapid development of endoscopic instruments and their widesprea
distribution to physicians who have not received formal supervised endo
scopic training has been associated with a proliferation of short courses o
gastrointestinal endoscopy. Such courses usually lack 'hands on' trainin
experience with patients; they are limited to didactic instruction and th
use of artificial models. Attendees of such courses are sometimes grante
certificates of attendance, and these, with or without supporting letters
are used by those applying for endoscopic privileges as sufficient evidenc
of competence to perform endoscopy. Privileges granted solely on the basi
of training in short courses do not assure patients that level of care to whic
they are entitled in today's medical community. If experience is acquire

utside a formal training program, it must be equivalent to that obtained
ithin such a program. Competence must be documented and skills
emonstrated.

lethods of granting hospital privileges to perform gastrointestinal ndoscopy

niform standards should be developed which apply equally to all hospital
aff requesting privileges to perform endoscopy, and to all areas where
1doscopy is performed within a given institution.

Privileges should be granted for each major category of endoscopy
:parately. The ability to perform one endoscopic procedure does not
nply adequate competency to perform another. Associated skills consi-
ered to be an integral part of an endoscopic category may be required
efore privileges for that category are granted. For example, competency
1 polypectomy and electrocoagulation must be documented before colon-
scopy privileges can be granted.

ndoscopic experience

he total time spent during training, learning and performing endoscopic
rocedures must be adequate for each major category for which privileges
re requested. These numbers should be regarded as a 'threshold'; i.e. the
1inimum number of supervised procedures required before it is possible
1at a trainee could have sufficient experience for certification (Table 1.2).
lowever, achieving the threshold number does not guarantee that the
ainee is competent to perform that procedure without supervision. That
ecision lies with the endoscopy training supervisor.

nformed consent for gastrointestinal endoscopy

)ver the last 30 years informed consent has undergone a transformation
om an ethical concept to a legal doctrine. Courts have recently begun to
nd physician liability based on the failure to obtain legally informed
onsent. The duty of all GI endoscopists is to obtain legally adequate
1formed consent before performing any endoscopic procedure on a
atient.

The crux of the Doctrine of Informed Consent is disclosure. The
lements of adequate disclosure include: (1) the nature of the proposed
rocedure; (2) the underlying reason why the procedure is necessary and
s goals; (3) the risks and complications of the procedure, including their
:lative incidence; and (4) reasonable alternatives to the proposed proc-
dure.

The endoscopist should be certain to explain the procedure to the
atient, including what will occur before, during and after the procedure.
he patient should be told why the procedure is necessary, and the

Table 1.2 Threshold for assessing competence

Procedures	Number of cases required
Standard	
Diagnostic EGD	100
Total Colonoscopy	100
Snare polypectomy	20
Non-variceal hemostasis (upper and lower; includes 10 active bleeders)	20*
Variceal hemostasis (includes 5 active bleeders)	15
Esophageal dilatation with guidewire	30
Flexible sigmoidoscopy	25
PEG	10
Advanced	
ERCP	100 (75 diagnostic; 25† therapeutic
Tumor ablation	20
Pneumatic dilatation for achalasia	5
Laparoscopy	25
Esophageal stent placement	10

* Included in total number.
† Includes 20 sphincterotomies and 5 stent placements and is in addition to the 75 diagnostic ERCP procedures.

anticipated benefits should be outlined. The risks and possible complica-tions of the procedure must be described. Not every possible risk o complication need be disclosed, but those which occur with significan frequency and those of a serious nature should be presented. If drugs are t be used, the endoscopist should include their hazards and risks. It i equally important to present the possible alternatives to the procedure including ones that may be more hazardous. If no alternatives exist, th patient should be so informed.

The endoscopist is best advised to obtain the patient's informed consen personally. This duty is not generally a delegatable one. The use o preprinted materials, diagrams and other audiovisual materials can b useful adjuncts to the patient's decision-making, but they are not sub stitutes for the physician–patient interaction. The patient should be give adequate time to deliberate and the endoscopist should solicit and answe questions.

Most hospitals require a formal writing such as a consent form to satisf their informed consent policies, although this writing is required by law i only a few States in the USA. The endoscopist must be mindful of the fac that informed consent is a process of disclosure and deliberation, no merely the signing of a form. The endoscopist should be certain t document that he or she obtained the patient's informed consent prior t the performance of a procedure.

There are four recognized exceptions to the legal Doctrine of Informe Consent: (1) the emergency exception, (2) incompetency, (3) therapeuti privilege, and (4) waiver. When there is inadequate time due to clinica

mergency and there is a threat to the patient's life, an endoscopist may
orgo obtaining the patient's informed consent. However, appropriate
fforts must be made to obtain consent from a relative before proceeding
under this exception. An incompetent patient cannot sufficiently parti-
ipate in the informed consent process. None the less, the endoscopist still
as a duty to obtain informed consent from that patient's legal guardian. In
eality, incompetency is no exception at all and is best viewed that way for
linical purposes. There are occasional patients who may be harmed by the
isclosure necessary to obtain informed consent. However, therapeutic
rivilege is probably overused by physicians, who overestimate the degree
o which patients will find disclosure disagreeable. Finally, a patient may
lect not to be told the elements of disclosure. In this circumstance, the
ndoscopist should be certain that the patient has full knowledge and
understanding of his or her right to informed consent and that he or she
oluntarily relinquishes it. Appropriate documentation is essential. Many
American hospitals have an office of 'Risk Management' that can advise in
ifficult cases. Regardless of the circumstances, the best interests of the
atient should always be the principal concern.

nfection control during gastrointestinal endoscopy

n spite of the large number and variety of GI procedures, documented
nstances of infectious complications remain exceedingly rare. Endoscopic
elated infections may occur in several situations.

> Organisms may be spread by contaminated equipment. Bacterial infections (e.g.
> *Salmonella, Pseudomonas*) have been acquired in this manner by patients
> undergoing endoscopy. Documented cases of endoscopic spread of viruses is
> either very rare, such as hepatitis B virus (HBV), or unreported, as with human
> immunodeficiency virus (HIV).
> Bacteria may spread during endoscopy from the GI tract through the blood-
> stream to potentially susceptible tissues or prostheses, possibly resulting in
> infection (e.g. bacterial endocarditis). (See below, Guidelines for antibiotic
> prophylaxis.)
> Patients with severe neutropenia, immune deficiency syndromes, or those
> receiving immunosuppressive chemotherapy may be at increased risk for endo-
> scopic transmission of disease.
> Infected patients may transmit disease to endoscopy personnel.

outine endoscopic cleaning and disinfection

he following are selected excerpts from the ASGE statement on endo-
copic cleaning and disinfection. The various techniques are described in
onsiderably greater detail in the unabridged guidelines.

leaning, sterilization and disinfection: definitions

> *Cleaning* is defined as the physical removal of organic material and/or soil from
> objects, usually using water with detergents designed to remove rather than kill
> organisms.

2 *Sterilization* is the act of killing all microbial life and the elimination of bacterial spores. It is most commonly done with heat or ethylene oxide gas.
3 *Disinfection* involves the killing of most microorganisms, including pathogens and is commonly done with the use of liquid germicides.

Mechanical cleaning

The first and most important step in the prevention of infection during endoscopy is mechanical cleaning. This should be done promptly after the use of endoscopes and accessories to avoid the formation of concretions. The insertion tube is cleaned with a sponge or cloth. The endoscope tip, biopsy ports (after removing the valves) and less accessible areas are cleaned with a cotton-tipped applicator. All endoscope channels should be brushed to remove particulate matter. Cleaning solution is suctioned or pumped through all channels. Endoscopic accessories are thoroughly cleaned with detergents and brushing of irregular surfaces. After mechanical cleaning, immersible equipment should be thoroughly rinsed with water. Non-immersible handles should be cleaned with alcohol-dampened cloths and towel dried.

Sterilization and disinfection

Cold gas (ethylene oxide) is effective for sterilizing flexible endoscopes but is impractical for routine use as it usually requires scheduling and up to 24 hours before reuse. *Autoclaving destroys flexible endoscopes.* Sterilization may be achieved by some liquid sterilants if the instrument is immersed completely for specified prolonged immersion periods. However, this procedure could severely damage flexible instruments. For instruments such as GI endoscopes which do not normally come into contact with sterile tissue, sterilization does not appear to be necessary for safe endoscopy. High-level disinfection with an Environmental Protection Agency (EPA) registered liquid sterilant/disinfectant is appropriate. Among the acceptable products, glutaraldehyde-based formulations are the most frequently used disinfectants for GI endoscopes. Exposure immersion times of 10 minutes are typically used and would appear to be sufficient to kill infectious agents likely to be encountered in GI endoscopy.

After each procedure, GI endoscopes should be thoroughly cleaned then soaked in a chemical sterilant/disinfectant according to the chemical manufacturer's directions and exposure time necessary to achieve disinfection. Following disinfection, endoscopic equipment must be rinsed free of residual germicide and dried. A tap water rinse of 30 seconds has been shown to remove glutaraldehyde effectively but residual odor may require a longer rinse and aeration time. Endoscopic accessories that may be heat stable (such as biopsy forceps) should be thoroughly cleaned. Certain accessories such as sphincterotomes, ERCP cannulas and sclerotherapy needles are disposed of or cleaned, dried and gas sterilized after use. The water bottle needs to be disinfected on a regular basis. Finally, it is mportant to have a properly designed environment for endoscope cleaning, with efficient venting of noxious fumes, etc.

Forced air drying and storage

A critical part of the cleaning and disinfection process involves forced air drying of the endoscope channels prior to storage. This process is important to prevent proliferation of residual bacteria and fungi during storage, and is even necessary following washing and disinfection in automated machines. It has been recommended that 70% alcohol be suctioned through all channels of ERCP endoscopes prior to forced air drying and storage. A sterile water or alcohol rinse should be performed prior to forced air drying and prolonged storage of endoscopes. Endoscopes should be stored hanging rather than in their boxes. Endoscopic washing machines may offer advantages such as automated washing and disinfection cycle times, freeing endoscopy assistants for other duties and reducing exposure to contaminated equipment and disinfectants. However, these machines may not assure a clean, disinfected endoscope and instances of contamination have been reported. It should be remembered that mechanical cleaning and brushing of the suction channels must be done prior to placing the endoscope in the washing machine.

Guidelines for antibiotic prophylaxis for GI procedures

Risk of bacteremia and endocarditis associated with endoscopic procedures

Bacterial endocarditis is a potentially life-threatening infection resulting from bacteremia in an individual with a susceptible cardiac lesion. Transient bacteremia may follow dental, endoscopic and surgical procedures. Other infections claimed to be a risk of bacteremia following endoscopic procedures include those involving prosthetic joints and vascular grafts. Antibiotic prophylaxis has been recommended for high-risk endoscopic procedures in patients with prosthetic heart valves, congenital cardiac malformations, rheumatic valvular disease, hypertrophic cardiomyopathy, prior history of bacterial endocarditis and mitral valve prolapse (MVP) with regurgitation (Table 1.3). Mitral valve prolapse is the most common lesion found in patients undergoing endoscopy, but only 20% of these have MVP with regurgitation. Cardiac conditions in which antibiotic prophylaxis is *not* recommended are listed in Table 1.4.

Bacteremia is a common occurrence which has been demonstrated after brushing teeth and chewing food. The frequency of bacteremia associated with endoscopic procedures is in the range 3–4%. The highest rates of bacteremia have been detected following esophageal dilatation and variceal sclerotherapy (as high as 54% and 18%, respectively). Transesophageal echocardiography (TEE) has been associated with bacteremia, as has laser therapy (around 30% incidence). As expected, the organisms

Table 1.3 Cardiac conditions for which endocarditis prophylaxis is recommended

Prosthetic cardiac valves (including prosthetic and homograft valves)
Previous bacterial endocarditis
Most congenital cardiac malformations
Rheumatic and other acquired valvular dysfunction, even after valvular
   surgery
Hypertrophic cardiomyopathy
Mitral valve prolapse with valvular regurgitation

(After American Heart Association, 1990)

Table 1.4 Cardiac conditions for which endocarditis prophylaxis is not recommended

Isolated secundum atrial septal defect
Surgical repair without residual defect beyond 6 months of secundum,
   atrial septal defect, ventricular septal defect, patent ductus arteriosus
Previous coronary artery bypass graft surgery
Physiologic, functional or innocent heart murmurs
Previous Kawasaki disease without valvular dysfunction
Mitral valve prolapse without valvular regurgitation

(After American Heart Association, 1990)

recovered from positive blood cultures vary depending on the site of the GI tract instrumented. Lower GI procedures (e.g. flexible sigmoidoscopy) are associated with bacteremia due to enteric organisms such as enterococcus, *Klebsiella* spp and *Escherichia coli*. In contrast, esophageal dilatation is most commonly associated with Gram-positive pathogens such as *Staphylococcus aureus* and *Streptococcus viridans*. It is worth stating that bacterial endocarditis related to endoscopy is *very uncommon*. Of the 15 cases so far reported, it has been suggested that only four are adequately documented.

Antibiotic prophylaxis

Although antibiotic prophylaxis has been recommended to prevent bacterial endocarditis, it is probable that most cases of endocarditis cannot be prevented in this way. However, this does not mean that patients with susceptible cardiac lesions undergoing high-risk endoscopic procedures should not be given antibiotics. The rationale for antibiotic prophylaxis assumes that it decreases the severity of bacteremia and the likelihood of bacterial adhesion to and growth on abnormal heart valves and prostheses. The hypothesis remains to be proved. Cases of bacterial endocarditis have occurred despite antibiotic prophylaxis, often after dental procedures.

    There are multiple factors involved in determining the efficacy of antibiotic prophylaxis, ranging from the choice of drug to the mode and iming of administration. For example, an antibiotic given shortly before a high-risk procedure may not reach bacteriostatic or bactericidal levels in the blood in time to prevent clinically significant bacteremia. Noting that the majority of cases of bacterial endocarditis reported to have followed GI procedures involved *Enterococcus faecalis*, the American Heart Association has recommended that prophylaxis be directed primarily against this organism. The standard prophylaxis regimen for GI procedures in high-risk patients includes parenteral (i.v. or i.m.) ampicillin or gentamicin before the procedure, followed by oral amoxicillin 6 hours after the initial dose (Table 1.5). An alternative oral regimen for low-risk patients is amoxicillin 3 g orally 1 hour before the procedure and 1.5 g 6 hours after the initial dose.

Prophylaxis for GI procedures is recommended for (1) sclerotherapy of esophageal varices, and (2) esophageal dilatation. Endocarditis prophylaxis is *not* recommended for endoscopy with or without biopsy with the following exception: 'In patients who have prosthetic heart valves, a previous history of endocarditis or surgically constructed systemic-pulmonary shunts, physicians may choose to administer prophylactic antibiotics even for low-risk procedures that involve the GI tract.'

Table 1.5 Antibiotic regimens for GI procedures

Drug	Dosage regimen
Standard regimen	
Ampicillin, gentamicin, amoxicillin	i.v. or i.m. ampicillin 2.0 g plus gentamicin 1.5 mg/kg (not to exceed 80 mg), 30 minutes before procedure; followed by amoxicillin, 1.5 g orally 6 hours after initial dose. Alternative: parenteral regimen may be repeated once 8 hours after initial dose
Penicillin allergy regimen	
Vancomycin, gentamicin	i.v. vancomycin 1.0 g over 1 hour plus i.v. or i.m. gentamicin, 1.5 mg/kg (not to exceed 80 mg), 1 hour before procedure; may be repeated once 8 hours after initial dose
Alternative low-risk patient regimen	
Oral amoxicillin	3.0 g orally 1 hour before procedure; then 1.5 g 6 hours after initial dose

(After American Heart Association, 1990)

Teaching aids: models and simulators

Endoscopic training tools

Most endoscopists regard themselves as experts on endoscopic training. However, the truth is that very little is understood about the process of acquiring endoscopic skills. Certainly, endoscopic training has changed little over the last 30 years, with one-to-one apprenticeship remaining the norm. Although this is certainly a time-honored way to teach endoscopy, it is demanding of expert endoscopists' time and may not be the most effective way for the novice to learn. A great variety of written and audiovisual materials are available to guide the trainee endoscopist, but there is no substitute for 'hands on' training with an endoscope. However, this often results in prolonged and uncomfortable procedures for patients being examined by trainees under supervision. Unfortunately, rubber and plastic models of the stomach and colon have proved to be a poor substitute for the real thing, and rarely maintain the interest of trainees. Recently, computerized training devices have been developed to simulate the experience of endoscopy without the use of patients (Figure 1.11). These simulations employ computer graphics or interactive video systems with control inputs provided through a highly modified 'dummy' endoscope. Simulation is a fledgling technology which has yet to be scientifically evaluated, however its proponents are confident that many of the basic hand–eye coordination skills required in GI endoscopy can be taught this way, sparing patients painful procedures and making the most effective use of supervised training by skilled endoscopists. Further development of simulation technology is awaited with interest.

Proctoring

A proctor acts as a monitor to evaluate the technical and cognitive skills of another physician. The proctor's position differs from that of a consultant or supervising instructor in that he or she does not directly participate in patient care, has no physician–patient relationship with the patient being

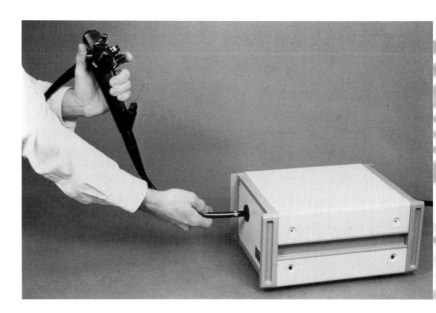

Figure 1.11 Endoscopic simulation training device. A highly modified dummy endoscope and a sophisticated 'black box' provide electrical inputs that drive a computer graphics simulation

reated, and does not receive a fee from the patient. A proctor represents he medical staff of a hospital or clinic and is responsible to the medical taff in connection with the credentialing of physicians seeking endoscopic rivileges. The ASGE has recently issued guidelines (Proctoring and Hospital Endoscopy Privileges) for the development of a proctoring policy within hospitals and clinics. These include:

Written guidelines

Guidelines must be carefully written and included in the hospital by-laws as n integral part of the credentialing process. Candidates for proctoring nclude initial applicants to the medical staff and for delineation of new linical privileges. Proctoring may also be appropriate for incumbent medical staff members who hold privileges for an endoscopic procedure but who have performed few over an extended period of time, or when a procedural technique changes in such a way that their prior training may no onger be adequate. In addition, proctoring may be one of several appropriate actions when a potential practice problem is identified by the hospital's quality assurance (QA) or risk management programs.

Proctoring is not a substitute for training and the proctor's function is to evaluate, not teach, the applicant. Comprehensive training in endoscopy must be acquired in an accredited program. An additional year of fellowship may be required of applicants seeking privileges to perform certain complex endoscopic procedures (e.g. ERCP with sphincterotomy). Graduates should have specific data from log books regarding the number of each procedure performed.

Qualifications of the proctor

The proctor should be a physician who holds the clinical privileges in the procedure being observed, and should possess sufficient expertise to judge the quality of care being rendered. The proctor should always be identified as a member or representative of a committe of the medical staff established as having responsibility for proctoring as one of its peer review functions. If no suitable proctor is available on the medical staff, outside experts should be recruited.

Ideally, each applicant for endoscopic privileges should be evaluated by more than one proctor. These proctors should be free of actual or perceived conflicts of interest which might create a bias against, or in favor of, the applicant.

The proctoring process

The proctor must engage in direct observation of the performance of endoscopic procedures over a specified period of time or for a specified number of cases. Although this may be coupled with retrospective review of cases, retrospective review cannot replace concurrent observation. The proctor should evaluate all aspects of the management of care in each case.

Individual circumstances will dictate which procedures require a formal proctoring process. Upper GI endoscopy (EGD), colonoscopy, polypectomy, esophageal dilatation, ERCP, percutaneous gastrostomy, flexible sigmoidoscopy and therapeutic use of the heater probe or laser are examples of techniques appropriate for proctoring. Diagnostic and therapeutic applications must be addressed separately.

The proctor should prepare a confidential written report for use by the credentials committee describing the type and number of cases observed and evaluating the applicant's performance. The proctor's report should be maintained in the applicant's credentials file and should be evaluated by the credentials committee at the time the applicant is considered for promotion from provision status.

The issue of whether and to what extent a proctor should intervene in a procedure is complex and unsettled. Certain situations may dictate that the proctor become a consultant to the applicant or actually intervene to assist in a procedure gone awry. If he or she goes beyond merely observing the procedure, the proctor has undertaken a duty of care to the patient which can result in liability arising from sequelae of the procedure. A proctor's involvement should be disclosed on the patient's chart and in the proctor's confidential report to the credentials committee. Potential legal problems can be ameliorated by having a formal, written protocol for proctoring and by maintaining detailed records.

Bibliography

General

Arrowsmith, J. B., Gerstman, B. B., Fleischer, D. E. and Benjamin, S. B. (1991) Results from the ASGE/US Food and Drug Administration Collaborative Study on Complication Rates and Drug Use during Gastrointestinal Endoscopy. *Gastrointestinal Endoscopy*, **37**, 421–427

ASGE Publications (booklets), available from ASGE, Thirteen Elm Street, Manchester, MA 01944:

Gastrointestinal Endoscopy: Diagnostic and Therapeutic Procedures. An Information Resource Manual
Guidelines for Establishment of Gastrointestinal Endoscopy Areas (revised August 1989)
Infection Control During Gastrointestinal Endoscopy (printed January 1988)
Informed Consent for Gastrointestinal Endoscopy (printed May 1986)
Methods of Granting Hospital Privileges to Perform Gastrointestinal Endoscopy (printed May 1986)
Monitoring of Patients Undergoing Gastrointestinal Endoscopic Procedures (printed August 1989)
Preparation of Patients for Gastrointestinal Endoscopy (printed January 1988)
Principles of Training in Gastrointestinal Endoscopy (printed May 1991)
Proctoring and Hospital Endoscopy Privileges (printed April 1981)

Standards of Practice of Gastrointestinal Endoscopy (revised March 1986)
Statement on Endoscopic Training (revised March 1986)
Statement on Role of Short Course in Endoscopic Training (reprinted March 1986)
The Role of Laparoscopy in the Diagnosis and Management of Gastrointestinal Disease (printed January 1988)
Tissue Sampling and Analysis (printed April 1981)

otton, P. B., Tytgat, G. N. J. and Williams, C. B. (eds) (1991) *Annual of Gastrointestinal Endoscopy*, Current Science Ltd, London.

oduced annually since 1988. An invaluable resource. Expert contributors assess the evious year's endoscopy-related publications, and provide an annotated bibliography. ghly recommended.

otton, P. B. and Williams, C. B. (1990) *Practical Gastrointestinal Endoscopy*, 3rd edn, Blackwell Scientific Publications, Oxford

rst published in 1980. Often cited as the 'gold standard' in endoscopy textbooks, by two ell-known endoscopists. Easy style, nice line drawings and a comprehensive bibliography. apter 10 begins with a concise review of the principles of electrosurgery. Highly commended.

unt, R. H. and Waye, J. D. (1981) *Colonoscopy: Techniques, Clinical Practice and Colour Atlas*, Chapman and Hall, London

lder text but full of useful tips by two expert colonoscopists.

eyers, W. C. and Scott Jones, R. (1990) *Textbook of Liver and Biliary Surgery*, J. B. Lippincott, Philadelphia

ew textbook that is a must for endoscopists who manage patients with hepatobiliary sorders.

hiller, K. F. R., Cockel, R. and Hunt, R. H. (1986) *A Colour Atlas of Gastrointestinal Endoscopy*, W. B. Saunders, Philadelphia

rst published in 1986. An older style atlas of fiberoptic photographs and X-rays. However, ntains much useful information and common sense.

vak, M. V. Jr. (ed.) (1987) *Gastroenterologic Endoscopy*, W. B. Saunders, Philadelphia

rst edition 1987. 1168 page multi-author textbook. Encyclopedic and therefore more for ference than casual reading. Excellent descriptions of endoscopic equipment, accessories, d special techniques.

aye, J., Geenen, J. E., Fleischer, D. and Venu, R. P. (1985) *Techniques in Therapeutic Endoscopy*, W. B. Saunders, Philadelphia

rst published 1987. By four distinguished American endoscopists. Profusely illustrated olor plates and diagrams). Emphasis on *therapeutic* endoscopy. Highly recommended.

aillie, J., Jowell, P., Evangelou, H., Bickel, W. and Cotton, P. (1991) Use of computer graphics simulation for teaching of flexible sigmoidoscopy. *Endoscopy*, **23**, 126–129

otoman, V. A. and Surawicz, C. M. (1986) Bacteremia with gastrointestinal procedures. *Gastrointestinal Endoscopy*, **32**, 342–345

e Knyrim, K., Seidlitz, H. Vakil, N. *et al.* (1990) Perspectives in 'electronic endoscopy'. *Endoscopy*, **22**, 2–8

leischer, D. (1989) Monitoring the patient receiving conscious sedation for gastrointestinal endoscopy: issues and guidelines. *Gastrointestinal Endoscopy*, **35**, 262–265

Meyer, G. W. (1991) Endocarditis prophylaxis for gastrointestinal procedures: rebuttal to the newest American Heart Association recommendations (editorial). *Gastrointestinal Endoscopy*, **37**, 201–202

Rosario, M. T. and Costa, N. F. (1990) Combination of midazolam and flumazeril in upper gastrointestinal endoscopy. *Gastrointestinal Endoscopy*, **36**, 30–33

Sivak, M. V. Jr. (1989) Endoscopic documentation — overview. *Annual of Gastrointestinal Endoscopy*, Current Science, London

Sivak, M. V. Jr. (1990) Privileges to perform endoscopy. *Gastrointestinal Endoscopy*, **36**, 73–74

Stroehlein, J. R., Barroso, A., Glombicki, A. and Sachs, I. (1990) Documentation of fluoroscopic and endoscopic images using a color video printer. *Gastrointestinal Endoscopy*, **36**, 392–394

Van Gossum, M., Seruys, L. E. and Cremer, M. (1989) Methods of disinfecting endoscopic material: results of an international survey. *Endoscopy*, **21**, 247–25

Wexler, R. M. (1989) Quality assurance: an overview and outline for gastrointestinal endoscopy. *American Journal of Gastroenterology*, **84**, 1482–1487

Wilcox, C. M., Forsmark, C. E. and Cello, J. P. (1990) Utility of droperidol for conscious sedation in gastrointestinal procedures. *Gastrointestinal Endoscopy*, **36**, 112–115

Williams, C. B., Baillie, J., Gillies, D. F., Borislow, D. and Cotton, P. B. (1990) Teaching gastrointestinal endoscopy by computer simulation: a prototype for colonoscopy and ERCP. *Gastrointestinal Endoscopy*, **36**, 49–54

2

Upper GI endoscopy

Most endoscopists begin their training with upper GI endoscopy, or esophagogastroduodenoscopy (EGD). Although this is generally regarded as the least difficult of the principal endoscopic procedures, that does not mean it is easy. However, once you become familiar with the equipment and techniques used in diagnostic and therapeutic EGD, the foundation for more complex procedures such as colonoscopy and ERCP has already been laid.

Endoscopes

There is a large variety of forward-viewing endoscopes available for EGD. In addition to the standard adult gastroscope there are small caliber (pediatric) instruments that are particularly useful in the presence of strictures and other anatomic abnormalities. At the other end of the spectrum, large channel therapeutic endoscopes are valuable when assessing patients with active GI bleeding. Oblique and side-viewing endoscopes have their place; specific indications will be pointed out. However, unless otherwise indicated our discussion of upper GI endoscopy will assume the use of standard forward-viewing instruments.

Indications and contraindications

Diagnostic EGD is generally indicated for evaluating:

Upper abdominal distress which persists despite an appropriate trial of therapy.
Upper abdominal distress associated with symptoms and/or signs suggesting serious organic disease (e.g. anorexia and weight loss).
Dysphagia or odynophagia.
Esophageal reflux symptoms which are persistent or recurrent despite appropriate therapy.
Persistent vomiting of unknown cause.
Other system disease in which the presence of upper GI (UGI) pathology might modify the planned management. Examples include patients with a history of GI bleeding who are scheduled for organ transplantation, long term anticoagulation or chronic non-steroidal therapy for arthritis.
Familial polyposis coli (for UGI screening).

8 X-ray findings of:
  (a) A suspected neoplastic lesion, for confirmation and specific histolog
      diagnosis.
  (b) Gastric or esophageal ulcer.
  (c) Evidence of upper tract stricture or obstruction.
9 Gastrointestinal bleeding:
  (a) In most actively bleeding patients.
  (b) When surgical therapy is contemplated.
  (c) When rebleeding occurs after acute self-limited blood loss.
  (d) When portal hypertension or aortoenteric fistula is suspected.
  (e) For presumed chronic blood loss and for iron deficiency anemia whe
      colonoscopy is negative.
10 When sampling of duodenal or jejunal tissue or fluid is indicated.

Diagnostic EGD is generally not indicated for evaluating:

1 Distress which is chronic, non-progressive, atypical for known organic diseas
  and is considered functional in origin (there are occasional exceptions in whic
  an endoscopic examination may be done once to rule out organic diseas
  especially if symptoms are unresponsive to therapy).
2 Uncomplicated heartburn responding to medical therapy.
3 Metastatic adenocarcinoma of unknown primary site when the results will n
  alter management.
4 X-ray findings of:
  (a) Asymptomatic or uncomplicated sliding hiatus hernia.
  (b) Uncomplicated duodenal bulb ulcer which has responded to therapy.
  (c) Deformed duodenal bulb when symptoms are absent or respond adequate
      to ulcer therapy.
5 Patients without GI symptoms about to undergo elective surgery for non-UC
  disease.

Sequential or periodic diagnostic EGD may be indicated:

1 In patients requiring periodic surveillance for proven Barrett's esophagus (
  familial polyposis coli.
2 For follow-up of selected esophageal, gastric or stomal ulcers to demonstra
  healing.
3 In patients with prior adenomatous gastric polyps.
4 Follow-up of adequacy of prior sclerotherapy of esophageal varices.

Sequential or periodic diagnostic EGD is generally not indicated for:

1 Surveillance for malignancy in patients with gastric atrophy, pernicious anemi
  treated achalasia or prior gastric operation.
2 Surveillance of healed benign disease such as esophagitis, or gastric or duoden
  ulcer.
3 Surveillance during chronic repeated dilatations of benign strictures unless the
  is a change in status.

Therapeutic EGD is generally indicated for:

1 Treatment of bleeding from lesions such as ulcers, tumors, vascular malforma
  tions (e.g. electrocoagulation, heater probe, laser photocoagulation or injectic
  therapy).

Sclerotherapy for bleeding from esophageal or proximal gastric varices.
Foreign body removal.
Removal of selected polypoid lesions.
Placement of feeding tubes (peroral, percutaneous endoscopic gastrostomy, percutaneous endoscopic jejunostomy).
Dilatation of stenotic lesions (e.g. with transendoscopic balloon dilators or dilating systems employing guidewires).
Palliative therapy of stenosing neoplasms (e.g. laser, bipolar electrocoagulation, stent placement).

Endoscopists must ensure that every procedure they do is appropriate. Procedures should never be done uncritically. The technical ability to perform an endoscopic procedure does not guarantee that it is safe and appropriate in every case. A GI endoscopist is a consultant who may be able to provide the safest and more effective diagnostic or therapeutic procedure once all the options have been assessed. An evaluation of these options is integral to the process of informed consent.

Contraindications

There are more relative than absolute contraindications to EGD.

Absolute contraindications

Known or suspected perforation of the GI tract.
Lack of adequately trained personnel to perform procedure.
Mentally competent patient refuses procedure after full explanation of options.
Lack of informed consent for non-urgent procedure.

Relative contraindications

Uncooperative or confused patient.
Unable to obtain informed consent (emergency exceptions exist).
Lack of necessary nursing/technical support and/or endoscopic equipment.
Patient ate food or antacids (or received enteral feeding) within 4 hours of procedure.
Unstable cardiac patient (e.g. recent myocardial infarction, unstable angina, untreated tachydysrhythmia, complete heart block).
Gross coagulopathy (e.g. platelets < 20 000 mm (20 × 10^9/liter), disseminated intravascular coagulation).
Unable to provide airway protection (endotracheal intubation) for endoscopy in patient with massive UGI bleeding.
High-grade intestinal obstruction.

Passing the endoscope

'Blind' passage of an endoscope is usually safe; the insertion tube is passed much like a mercury dilator, with the patient being encouraged to swallow. However, there are several limitations of this technique. First, the

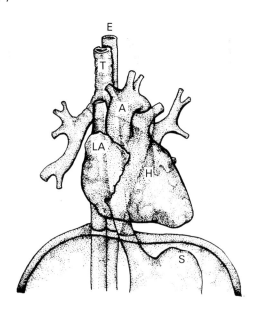

Figure 2.1 The esophagus and its anatomical relations. E, esophagus; T, trachea; A, thoracic aorta; LA, left atrium; H, heart; S, stomach

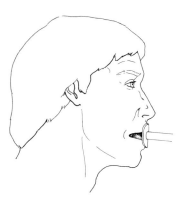

Figure 2.2 Patient with mouthpiece in position

endoscopist may not appreciate problematic anatomy, e.g. a pharyngeal pouch (Zenker's diverticulum) or an esophageal stricture, before encountering resistance. Second, unless a particularly thorough inspection is made at the end of the procedure (on withdrawing the endoscope), the hypopharynx will not be seen. Inspection of the vocal cords, piriform recesses and adjacent structures should be part of every EGD, as incidental pathology in the pharynx and upper larynx may be discovered.

Trainee endoscopists should learn to pass the endoscope *under direct vision*. This technique not only allows inspection of the hypopharynx, but ensures that the endoscope is positioned correctly for esophageal intubation. Using direct vision, the risk of inadvertent laryngeal intubation is much reduced. Difficult or unusual pharyngeal and esophageal anatomy can be identified before mechanical resistance is encountered.

The upper esophageal sphincter is located approximately 15–18 cm from the lips. Externally it is at the level of the thyroid cartilage. It is important to know the anatomical relationships of the esophagus within the thorax (Figure 2.1). The upper esophageal sphincter will usually open if the patient attempts to swallow. However, when the throat has been numbed by local anesthetic and intravenous sedation given, a patient may not be able to cooperate. Placing the tip of the endoscope at the introitus and applying *gentle* pressure will encourage the sphincter to open. Passing an endoscope under direct vision is undoubtedly a more difficult technique to master than the 'blind' technique but it is well worth the effort. Before getting into technicalities, a few words about 'setting the scene'. The patient should lie comfortably in the left lateral position with a mouth guard (Figure 2.2) (or bite piece) held gently between the teeth (or gums). Mouth guards should be used routinely: even deeply sedated patients can bite and edentulous jaws exert surprisingly large forces. If topical anestheia has been given, assess its effect. Touch the back of the throat with a gloved finger or tongue blade; if the patient gags, repeat the application. Intravenous sedation should render the patient drowsy but easily rousable.

A few words of explanation and encouragement at each stage of the procedure will allay anxiety. Making patients feel that they have an active role in helping with the procedure is good psychology.

After checking that the endoscope is fully functional (see Chapter 1, Endoscopes and accessories), you are ready to start. The endoscope is passed over the back of the tongue with downward angulation of the tip (Figure 2.3). As the view at this point is limited it is important to keep close to the midline. The uvula is a useful anatomic landmark; however, as it is easily traumatized by the endoscope, pass the uvula on one side or the other. The next landmark is the epiglottis (Figure 2.4). From the endoscopic perspective, one aims downwards (the 6 o'clock position) to reach the posterior hypopharynx. Figure 2.5 shows the esophageal introitus with surrounding structures, including the aryepiglottic folds and vocal cords. Although the upper esophageal sphincter sometimes opens in a directly posterior position, it is usually more effective to place the tip of the endoscope on one side or the other to look for the opening.

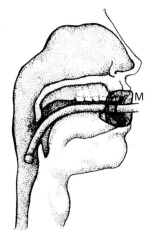

Figure 2.3 Endoscope passed into hypopharynx. Mouthpiece (M) in position

How much pressure you can safely apply while trying to coax the upper esophageal sphincter to open is learned by experience. Certainly, excessive force risks perforation. If the sphincter does not open with mild to moderate pressure over the orifice, withdraw a little and start again. Sometimes moving to the opposite piriform recess works. What can be done if repeated attempts to pass the endoscope under direct vision fail? Sometimes it may be easier to pass the instrument 'blindly', making use of the swallowing mechanism. Another option is to use an endoscope with a smaller external diameter, such as a pediatric gastroscope. These instruments are not routinely used for endoscopy in adults because of their limitations: they can be difficult to advance through a tight pylorus, due to extreme flexibility, and they have a small instrument channel, limiting the size of biopsies that can be taken. Another technique worth trying when intubation proves difficult is passage of a small mercury bougie (e.g. Maloney dilator). If this can be swallowed with ease the endoscope is reintroduced and will frequently pass without further difficulty. If these 'tricks' fail, it is appropriate to ask a more experienced endoscopist to assess the situation. Finally, if there appears to be a significant obstruction to endoscope passage, the procedure should be abandoned and a radiologic contrast study obtained to define the relevant anatomy.

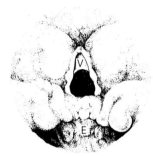

Figure 2.4 Hypopharynx (endoscopic view). V, vocal cords; E, epiglottis

A pharyngeal (Zenker's) diverticulum characteristically arises just below the upper esophageal sphincter, more often on the left side. This abnormality usually makes it difficult to pass an endoscope 'blind'. Under direct vision, it is obvious that the endoscope is passing into a blind-ending pouch. Once the problem has been identified, careful inspection of the neck of the pouch will usually reveal the true opening into the esophagus.

The upper esophageal sphincter may prove an impediment to the recovery of ingested foreign bodies. When a therapeutic procedure such as foreign body retrieval is being considered, it can be helpful to pass an

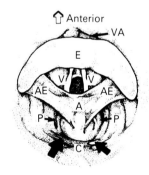

Figure 2.5 Hypopharyngeal endoscopic anatomy. E, epiglottis; A, arytenoid; AE, aryepiglottic folds; P, piriform recesses; VA, Vallecula; V, vocal cords; C, cricopharyngeus

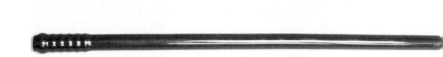

Figure 2.6 Endoscope overtube

overtube into the esophagus (Figure 2.6). The tube keeps the sphincter open, allowing endoscopes to be advanced and withdrawn repeatedly without resistance. It also provides valuable protection to the airway which is especially at risk during foreign body removal and endoscopic treatment of active UGI bleeding.

Examining the esophagus

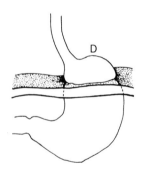

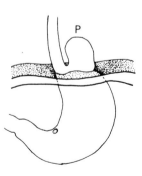

Figure 2.7 The two principal types of hiatus hernia: direct (D) and paraesophageal (P)

As the esophagus is a long, thin tube, an endoscope tends to stay in the axis of the lumen, which maintains a forward view during insertion and withdrawal. In the partially decompressed esophagus longitudinal folds are noted, although when distended with air it may appear rather featureless. On the way down, left atrial and/or aortic pulsation may be seen, especially in the elderly. In normal adults, the gastroesophageal junction lies approximately 40 cm from the lips. Although the exact measurement varies between individuals it is remarkably constant, with usually no more than about 2 cm variation above or below the 40 cm mark. There are several clues to the exact location of the gastroesophageal junction. First, there is loss of the esophageal subepithelial vascular pattern as the endoscope passes into the stomach, which has a columnar-type epithelium. A particularly important anatomic landmark is the so-called Z-line. This irregular, circumferential ridge that marks the anatomic border between the esophagus and the stomach is the squamocolumnar junction. This area is particularly important in patients with Barrett's esophagus, where the Z-line migrates up into the esophagus. The gastroesophageal junction is related to the diaphragmatic hiatus. This relationship is inconstant, particularly if the patient has upward herniation of the stomach into the chest (a hiatus hernia). The location of the diaphragmatic hiatus can be detected by observing pinching of the esophagus which occurs when the patient is asked to sniff. There are two types of hiatus hernia: direct (or 'sliding') and paraesophageal (Figure 2.7). The direct hiatus hernia is straightforward to detect, particularly if the sniff test is used. In a paraesophageal hernia, the gastroesophageal junction usually remains in its expected position. The hernia is actually above the level of the junction and may provide difficulty in orientation, especially for the novice endoscopist.

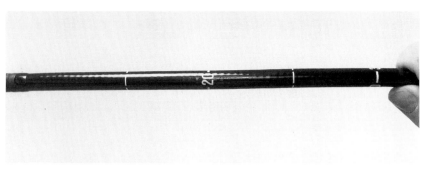

Figure 2.8 Insertion tube markings

It is important to document the level of esophageal lesions. Endoscopy provides a useful reference for the radiologist and surgeon. If pathology is seen its location should be recorded accurately (e.g. 'exophytic mass on the posterior wall from 28–30 cm from the lips'). As the endoscope is essentially straight within the esophagus, distances from the lips or teeth can be read from external markings on the outer plastic sheath. Standard gastroscopes are usually marked in 5 cm increments (Figure 2.8).

Examining the stomach

The histologic areas of the stomach (cardia, fundus, body and antrum) do not have instantly recognizable boundaries at endoscopy. However, there are some useful landmarks. The stomach is normally a deflated sac when the endoscope is first introduced. It is a common mistake to attempt to fully inflate the stomach at the start. This is uncomfortable for the patient, who will often belch or retch. If there is a large pool of fluid in the gastric fundus, try to remove this but take care to avoid creating mucosal suction artifacts. To aspirate fluid, position the endoscope tip just above the surface of the pool, rather than under it (Figure 2.9). This reduces the risk of sucking mucosa against the tip of the endoscope, which produces a red mark.

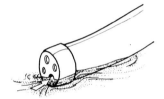

Figure 2.9 To aspirate fluid, position 'scope tip at or above the surface

Once in the fundus, look around and orient yourself. Air insufflation should be limited initially to what is required to obtain a lumenal view. Rather than trying to achieve a complete examination of the stomach before inspecting the duodenum, it is probably wise to head for the pylorus from the start. However, do look around while moving towards the pylorus; this may be the only view of virgin mucosa before endoscope artifacts are created. The shortest route to the pylorus is along the lesser curvature. It is good practice to follow the lesser curvature, using the minimum insufflation necessary to maintain a view. However, the endoscope will try to follow the greater curvature of the stomach (Figure 2.10). This can be a particularly long route, especially in the so-called J-shaped stomach; a straightening maneuver may be required to advance into and beyond the duodenal bulb. Locating the pylorus and negotiating the pyloric channel is often a challenge to the novice. However, by using clues from the mucosal fold pattern and the propagation of peristaltic waves, it is

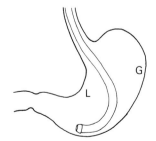

Figure 2.10 Endoscope tends to follow greater curvature (G) of the stomach. L, lesser curvature

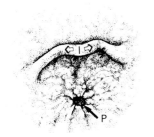

Figure 2.11 The incisura angularis (I) and pylorus (P)

almost always possible to identify the pylorus. There is a way out of almost every stomach, so be persistent.

Visualizing gastric anatomy from the fundus with a patient in the left lateral position, the endoscopist sees the following: the lesser curvature in the 12 o'clock (up) position and the greater curvature at 6 o'clock (down). Gravity causes fluid to pool in the dependent part of the stomach. If aspiration fails to clear this fluid, the hidden mucosa can be exposed by turning the patient 90° (i.e. prone or supine). The angulus (or incisura angularis) is a useful landmark (Figure 2.11) located approximately two-thirds of the way down the lesser curvature between the gastroesophageal junction and the pylorus. It appears as a transverse ridge. A good view of this area is imporant, as the angulus is a common site for gastric ulcers. There is a tongue of antral mucosa that extends up the lesser curvature almost to the gastroesophageal junction. This mucosa is particularly susceptible to ulceration.

When difficulty is encountered locating the pylorus, first find the angulus then follow the sweep of the antrum to the gastric outlet. The rugal folds of the fundus and body give way to the smooth mucosa of the antrum. The gastric rugae are pliable, have a rather velvety texture and appear darker than the flat, reflective antral mucosa.

Retroflexion

A gastric retroflexion maneuver can be performed either before inspecting the duodenum or afterwards. This is largely a matter of personal preference. However, as it may become progressively more difficult to intubate the pylorus and duodenum as sedation wears off and the patient becomes less cooperative, plan to examine these areas at the earliest opportunity. Retroflexion makes inspection of otherwise inaccessible areas, e.g. the cardia, fundus, gastroesophageal junction and proximal lesser curvature, straightforward. This maneuver takes advantage of the extreme flexibility of the endoscope tip. An adequate retroflexed view requires a degree of gastric distension; this is difficult to achieve when a patient persistently belches up air during endoscopy.

The most satisfactory starting position for retroflexion has the endoscope lying along the greater curvature with the tip well down in the gastric antrum. The tip is then rotated 'up' using the up–down control wheel, which can be operated by the thumb of the hand holding the endoscope (Figure 2.12). During retroflexion, the angulus comes into view first, then the lesser curvature leading up to the fundus and gastroesophageal junction (Figure 2.13). With full upward deflection of the endoscope tip, the shaft of the insertion tube should be clearly visible (Figure 2.14). It may be helpful to lock the control wheels in position. With the tip of the endoscope retroflexed, you need to withdraw for the endoscopic view to advance. A rotatory motion around the endoscope axis during gentle withdrawal will obtain a 360° view. Appropriate insertion, withdrawal and torsion in the long axis of the endoscope should achieve visualization of the entire gastric

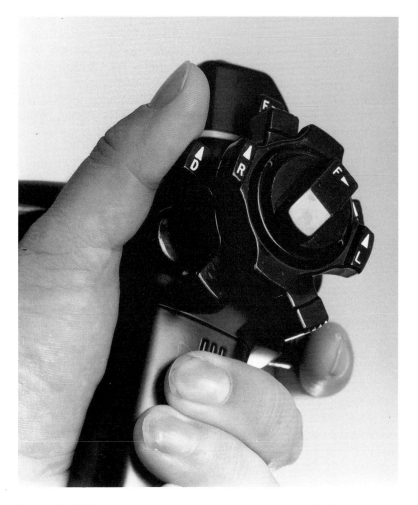

Figure 2.12 Thumb used to manipulate up–down control

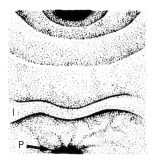

Figure 2.13 The incisura angularis (I) is a prominent landmark on the way to the pylorus (P). The lesser curve extends proximal to the incisura towards the gastroesophageal junction

fundus. It is appropriate to mention here that it may be difficult or impossible to pass biopsy forceps and other accessories when the tip of the endoscope is retroflexed. Never use force against resistance in this situation, as the endoscope may be damaged. To pass biopsy forceps, it may be necessary to partially or completely release the controls maintaining retroflexion. Once the instrument has advanced beyond the tip, i.e. comes into endoscopic view, the endoscope can be retroflexed again. Although it is technically possible to withdraw a retroflexed endoscope into a hiatus hernia, or even the distal esophagus, this should be done with great care, if at all, as it is possible to get stuck. Should this happen, insufflate to distend the esophagus or stomach, then gently push. If resistance continues, this maneuver should be repeated with the aid of fluoroscopy.

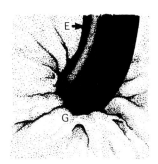

Figure 2.14 Retroflexion in the fundus reveals the endoscope (E) insertion tube passing through the gastroesophageal junction (G)

The postsurgical stomach

Postsurgical stomach anatomy offers challenges to every endoscopist, regardless of experience. The gastric remnant is often small and difficult to maintain inflated due to the enlarged outlet. Operations performed for gastric and duodenal ulcers include partial gastrectomy with Billroth I and II anastomoses, pyloroplasty and standard gastroenterostomy. In addition, a variety of gastroplasty procedures are performed to assist weight reduction. Working out the anatomy of a surgically altered stomach is a test of intellect and problem-solving ability. With experience, the postsurgical stomach becomes a familiar and less disorienting environment (see below, Problems).

Pylorus and duodenum

The pylorus is a short channel connecting the gastric antrum to the duodenum. It has an important role in digestion, metering the volume of food delivered to the duodenum for further breakdown and absorption. The pylorus has intrinsic muscular activity, acting like a valve. The opening and closing of the normal pylorus is synchronized with gastric antral peristalsis. If the pylorus cannot easily be identified, antral peristaltic waves will lead you there. The immediate prepyloric area merits close inspection, as this is a common site for erosions and ulcers. The pylorus can be difficult to intubate, especially when the endoscope tip is in a mechanically unfavorable position, e.g. when the stomach is long and J-shaped. Small, coordinated movements are needed to maintain station 'over' the pylorus. If it will not yield to forward pressure, simultaneous air insufflation often persuades the pylorus to open. An unduly spastic pylorus may indicate the presence of a 'channel ulcer'. For this reason, it is important to inspect the pyloric channel; the best view is obtained on withdrawing the endoscope. Spasm of the pylorus must be distinguished from stenosis, usually the result of peptic ulceration. If the pylorus is severely stenosed, endoscopic balloon dilatation may be necessary to gain access to the duodenum. Following chronic ulceration, the pylorus may assume an irregular shape. Surgical widening of the pylorus (pyloroplasty) usually leaves a gaping and easily intubated orifice.

The duodenum is described as having four parts; the third and fourth are beyond the reach of standard gastroscopes. The first part is commonly referred to as the *duodenal bulb*. It is fortunate for endoscopists that the vast majority of duodenal ulcers occur in the bulb. The anterior wall of the bulb, which as a rule does not contain mucosal folds, is the first view seen after intubating the pylorus. From the endoscopist's perspective, the bulbar duodenum takes a right turn; anatomically, this turn is posterior. Where the first (D1) and second (D2) parts of duodenum meet, there is a further right turn as the duodenum descends inferiorly (or caudally). This area may be blind to the endoscopist during insertion of the endoscope. D2 is recongizable by the appearance of circular rings, the valvulae conni-ventes.

When D2 is entered, the endoscope is usually in the long position (Figure 2.15), with a loop of insertion tube in the stomach. On withdrawal, the instrument will straighten, causing the tip to advance (Figure 2.16). The strange combination of the endoscopic view advancing while the instrument is withdrawn is called *paradoxical motion*. As described in Chapter 4, this straightening maneuver is important to endoscopic retro-grade cholangiopancreatography (ERCP). The duodenum is easier to inspect as the endoscope is withdrawn in its straightened position. However, the endoscope tends to fall out of the duodenum (into the stomach) in the straightened position, even when withdrawal is carefully controlled. For this reason, repeated duodenal intubation and inspection may be necessary to insure an adequate examination. The posterior wall of distal D1 and the D1–D2 junction often remain hidden from view. Unfortunately, as the field of view of a duodenoscope points medially, this instrument rarely adds useful information about posterior D1 and D2 lesions. Finally, no matter how good you think the view is, the main and accessory duodenal papillae cannot be inspected completely with a forward-viewing endoscope. If papillary pathology is suspected, the medial wall of D2 should be examined using a side-viewing duodenoscope.

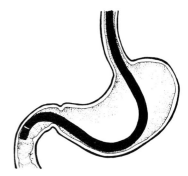

Figure 2.15 Endoscope in 'long' position in the duodenum

Increasing diagnostic yield: biopsies, brushings and aspirates

Obtaining specimens for histologic, cytologic and microbiologic analysis is an important role of endoscopy. To maximize diagnostic yield, material must be taken from the most favorable site and sent to the laboratory in an appropriate transport medium, accompanied by a request form providing (1) a brief clinical history, (2) the suspected diagnosis, and (3) the examination requested. Most laboratories appreciate advance warning if other than routine processing is needed (e.g. immunoperoxidase staining, culture for atypical mycobacteria). A telephone call to the laboratory to discuss your request and ascertain their requirements will avert most handling problems.

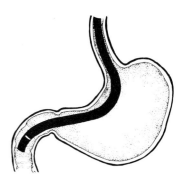

Figure 2.16 Straighten 'scope on withdrawal

Biopsies

A biopsy is a sample of tissue taken to determine the presence or absence of disease. Biopsy forceps used by endoscopists come in all shapes and sizes (see Figure 1.7). For all but the smallest lesions, multiple biopsies are preferred to increase diagnostic yield. A sliding handle is used to open and close biopsy forceps. To pass through the instrument channel of an endoscope forceps must be closed. When the lesion to be biopsied is clearly visible, the forceps are opened and applied firmly at the desired site. The forceps are then closed and the biopsy removed with a tug. This process is repeated until the desired number of biopises have been obtained.

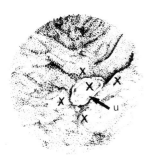

Figure 2.17 Preferred sites for biopsy of an ulcer (U): the base and in each quadrant around the growing edge

When taking biopsies from a gastric or esophageal ulcer to look for malignancy, at least one should be taken from each quadrant of the ulcer and two from the base (Figure 2.17). The growing edge of an ulcer is the best place to look for abnormal mitotic activity characteristic of malignancy. Submucosal masses present particular difficulty, as superficial biopsies show only normal mucosa. One way to gain access to a submucosal mass is repeated biopsy in the same place. However, tunneling, as this technique is called, should be avoided where the bowel wall is thin or inflamed.

If a submucosal mass is sufficiently prominent, part of it can be removed using snare electrocautery and retrieved for histologic examination. A soft and fluctuant submucosal mass in the distal esophagus or gastric fundus may be a solitary varix. Biopsy or snare electrocautery of a varix will cause impressive bleeding, which may be catastrophic. For this reason, do not biopsy any lesion that could be a varix.

It helps processing of biopsies to mount them on a flat surface. A small square of cardboard or even a slice of cucumber can be used. Although pathologists like to have biopsies oriented with the mucosa upwards, it is almost impossible to achieve this with standard endoscopic biopsy specimens.

If endoscopic biopsies of the distal duodenum have been taken to look for the protozoan parasite *Giardia lamblia*, it is useful to make a smear preparation of biopsy mucus on a cytology slide. Impale a biopsy specimen on the tip of a hypodermic needle and run it back and forth along the surface of a slide, which is then prepared for cytologic examination. A smear preparation occasionally yields a positive indentification of *G. lamblia*.

Brushings

Endoscopic brushings provide an additional opportunity to diagnose malignancy and are helpful in identifying candidiasis (thrush) and certain viral infections (e.g. cytomegalovirus). The bristles of an endoscopic brush are on the end of a wire that can be moved in and out of a plastic sleeve (see Figure 1.8). Repeated brushings are taken tangential to the lesion, then the brush is pulled back into its sleeve before withdrawing it from the endoscope. The material on the bristles is used to make smear preparations on several slides, which are air dried and sprayed with fixative, where appropriate.

Salvage cytology can increase diagnostic yield. There are two techniques: (1) the used cytology brush is agitated vigorously in a container of saline or water, which is then centrifuged and any precipitate is stained for cytologic examination; or (2) after the endoscopy, fluid sucked through the instrument channel is collected in a trap and sent for similar processing.

Aspirates

Fluid collected at endoscopy (e.g. duodenal aspirate, bile, pancreatic juice) can be used for both cytologic and microbiologic examination. To avoid contamination from debris in the instrument channel, fluid should be aspirated through a catheter into a syringe or clean container (trap). Bile may be sent for anaerobic culture if it is collected appropriately.

Helicobacter pylori

Helicobacter pylori is believed to be the cause of chronic peptic ulceration in certain patients refractory to H_2-blocker therapy. Clinically significant colonization with *H. pylori* may be diagnosed by histologic examination and bacteriologic culture of gastric antral biopsies. There is currently a vogue for rapid diagnosis kits that can be used in the endoscopy suite. These kits use chemical indicators to detect the urease activity of *H. pylori*. Fresh endoscopic biopsies are placed on a gel containing urea and the chemical indicator. The presence of *H. pylori* is indicated by a color change when urea is broken down into ammonia.

Problems

Agitation

Patients may become agitated during endoscopy for a variety of reasons. If the cause cannot be identified and remedied easily, the procedure should be stopped. If endoscopy is prolonged, extra sedation may be needed. However, the temptation to repeatedly 'top up' sedation as a patient becomes increasingly agitated should be resisted. If agitation is due to pain, the patient may become rapidly over-sedated when the procedure stops; automatic excitation that maintains consciousness disappears and deep sedation, even apnea, can ensue within seconds. Patients who regularly use benzodiazepines or narcotic analgesics are particularly difficult to sedate, due to acquired tolerance. Intravenous diazepam may disinhibit or cause paradoxical excitation in those who habitually use alcohol. The pulse oximeter is valuable for monitoring conscious sedation: a fall in arterial oxygen saturation often precedes clinical evidence of respiratory depression.

Over-sedation

The choice of intravenous sedation is less important than your familiarity with the drugs and their effect. Great care is required when changing over to a new agent. All intravenous sedatives should be titrated slowly against patient response. It is particularly dangerous to give any benzodiazepine (e.g. diazepam, midazolam), droperidol or fentanyl by bolus injection, especially in the elderly who may require very small doses. The specific narcotic antagonist, naloxone (Narcan), will reverse the effects of meperidine (pethidine; Demerol) and other narcotic sedatives, but not completely as naloxone is a weak narcotic itself. As intravenous naloxone has a short duration of action, it is useful to give an intramuscular dose simultaneously. A specific benzodiazepine antagonist, flumazenil, has been developed and is available in Europe, but not (at the time of writing) in the USA. Flumazenil is reported to be very effective; however, at present it is too expensive to use routinely after endoscopy to reverse benzodiazepine sedation.

Until flumazenil or one of its derivatives becomes available in the USA, respiratory depression caused by benzodiazepines will continue to be managed there by ventilatory support until spontaneous respiration is restored. (For further discussion of Conscious sedation, see Chapter 1.)

Getting lost

A cardinal rule of all endoscopy is that when unsure of location, withdraw. Inexperienced endoscopists may lose their way in a pharyngeal diverticulum, a large hiatus hernia or in the postsurgical stomach. A common cause of being uncertain of position is failure to maintain a lumenal view. When the endoscope tip is very close to mucosa, all that can be seen is the reflection from transilluminated bowel wall: a 'red out'. If the endoscope is then advanced against resistance, pressure on the bowel wall and its vasculature causes blanching: a 'white out'. Experienced endoscopists develop spatial awareness and a 'feel' for the pressure being applied; they can accept brief loss of lumenal view during certain maneuvers (e.g. 'slide by' technique for colonoscopy). However, as a general rule, the immediate response to a 'red out' or 'white out' should be to withdraw the endoscope to restore the lumenal view.

When air insufflation is inadequate, either due to equipment failure or a patient's inability to retain air, the endoscopic view will be suboptimal. A faulty or inoperative air pump should be identified before the procedure starts if a pre-endoscopy check-list is followed.

A pharyngeal pouch (Zenker's diverticulum) can make intubation difficult but the problem should be recognized if the endoscope is passed under direct vision. An upper GI contrast study (barium esophagram) is valuable for evaluating patients with dysphagia or regurgitation; diverticula, webs and strictures can be identified before they cause problems during endoscopy.

The postsurgical stomach lacks normal landmarks and is difficult to keep inflated. A food bezoar may be present due to loss of gastric motility. If a gastroenterostomy is present, the stoma should be identified and examined. It can be difficult to decide which limb (afferent or efferent) of a Billroth II anastomosis has been entered; sometimes fluoroscopy can help. If you reach a blind ending or see the duodenal papilla, you are in the fferent limb (Figure 2.18). To avoid repeatedly entering a limb that has lready been examined, take a mucosal biopsy about 15 cm from the toma; this produces a harmless but easily recognized bleeding site. Using dye like methylene blue to mark the afferent limb seems a good idea. Iowever, motility carries dye back up the afferent limb into the efferent imb as well as into the gastric remnant, turning everything blue and adding o the confusion!

Retained food limits the endoscopic view. If the patient has genuinely asted overnight, or for a minimum of 4 hours before the procedure, gastric etention suggests either a motility problem or gastric outlet obstruction. If ood, or a bezoar, seriously obscures the endoscopic view there are two ptions: (1) abandon the procedure and reschedule for a later date, or (2) emove the endoscope, lavage the stomach through a large bore tube, then epeat the endoscopy. Do not attempt to suck food debris through the ndoscope: this will quickly block the suction channel. When motility is eriously disordered, e.g. in diabetics and chronic renal failure patients vith gastroparesis, food may remain in the stomach for long periods. Repeated gastric lavage may be necessary to prepare these patients for ndoscopy, as prokinetic agents (e.g. metoclopramide) rarely help. Similar aveats apply in patients with long-standing achalasia; the chronically lilated esophagus may be full of retained food and secretions.

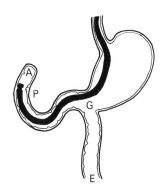

Figure 2.18 Billroth II anatomy. A, blind-ending afferent (duodenal) limb; P, papilla; G, gastroenterostomy; E, efferent limb

ncountering resistance

although primarily a discussion about strictures, the following comments pply equally to webs and pyloric stenosis. A significant stricture provides esistance to advancing the endoscope. As the external diameter of an dult gastroscope is about 11 mm, any fixed narrowing smaller than this auses a problem. An endoscope should *never* be used as a blunt dilator. If pediatric gastroscope is available, it may be possible to advance beyond he stricture. An endoscopist with the necessary training and experience nay then choose to leave a guidewire through an esophageal stricture to acilitate the passage of dilators (e.g. Savary) under fluoroscopy. An lternative way to dilate a stricture (including pyloric stenosis) is to use a hrough-the-'scope (TTS) dilating balloon. Stricture dilatation is discussed n more detail below (Basic therapeutics in the upper GI tract).

omplications

omplications of upper GI endoscopy include those related to medication e.g. allergy, thrombophlebitis), bleeding and perforation.

Bleeding following mucosal biopsy is rarely of clinical significance. Iowever, dramatic hemorrhage may follow inadvertent biopsy of an sophageal, gastric or duodenal varix. Coagulopathy, due to a low platelet ount (e.g. $< 20\ 000/mm^3$ (20×10^9/litre)), gross prolongation of the rothrombin time, specific clotting factor deficiency (e.g. hemophilia) or therapeutic anticoagulation, is a relative contraindication to endoscopy and, for all but the most fearless, an absolute contraindication to endoscopic biopsy. If endoscopic biopsy or a therapeutic procedure (e.g. stricture dilatation, endoscopic sphincterotomy) is unavoidable, temporary correction of the coagulopathy by transfusion of platelets, fresh frozen plasma or clotting factors or withholding anticoagulants will reduce the immediate risks. However, delayed hemorrhage may still occur. Patients who regularly use aspirin and non-steroidal anti-inflammatory drugs (NSAIDs) (e.g. indomethacin) are likely to have a prolonged bleeding time. It takes about 1 week for normal platelet adhesiveness to be restored after stopping these drugs. Prolongation of the bleeding time rarely causes problems after simple biopsy but it is a wise precaution to stop aspirin and NSAIDs 1 week before elective polypectomy or duodenal sphincterotomy. Patients on long-term oral anticoagulation may have to be admitted to hospital for temporary conversion to intravenous heparin in preparation for biopsy or a therapeutic procedure. As heparin has a short half-life in the circulation, normal coagulation can be restored by stopping heparin infusion 4–6 hours before the procedure. Anticoagulation can be reinstituted a few hours later with little risk of bleeding. As biopsy carries increased risks for severely immunocompromised patients, mucosal brushings offer a useful alternative in the evaluation of opportunistic infection, such as candidiasis and viral esophagitis. *Note that invasive candidiasis cannot be confirmed by brushings only.*

Endoscopic methods of hemostasis can be used to treat iatrogenic bleeding. These techniques are discussed below (Basic therapeutics in the upper GI tract).

Perforation of a viscus during endoscopy is a rare but invariably serious complication which can be life threatening in the elderly and debilitated. Perforation is an acknowledged risk of certain therapeutic procedures such as laser ablation and endoscopic stenting of obstructing tumors. However, this risk is calculated; for patients with inoperable malignancy an endoscopic procedure may offer the only chance of palliation. It is of great concern when a perforation occurs in the absence of gut pathology. Most of these perforations could be avoided by observing some basic rules of endoscopy: pass the endoscope under direct vision, don't advance when you can't see, don't keep pushing against resistance, never use an endoscope as a blunt dilator and never pass a dilator over a guidewire if you are unsure of its position.

A perforation may be recognized when it happens, or soon afterwards when the patient develops signs and symptoms of mediastinal, peritoneal or retroperitoneal irritation. If a perforation is suspected during endoscopy, the procedure should be discontinued immediately. The patient should have nothing by mouth and, except in esophageal injury, a nasogastric tube should be placed for gastric suction. Although plain radiograms showing free mediastinal, peritoneal or retroperitoneal air leave no doubt that a perforation has occurred, a contrast study may be necessary to pin-point the site of injury. A water-soluble contrast agent such as Gastrografin should be used instead of barium, which is irritant to

leural surfaces and the peritoneum. Provide intravenous fluids (as the
atient cannot drink) and start parenteral broad spectrum antibiotics. A
anagement plan should be formulated with the surgeon who will operate
needed. All parties must agree on indicators for surgical intervention,
g. worsening fever despite parenteral antibiotics, abscess formation, etc.
urgery may be avoided if pleural effusions and abdominal abscesses can
e drained percutaneously. However, perforations that fail to seal off
ontaneously often require surgical repair.

The morbidity and mortality of endoscopic perforations are increased by
elay; early recognition and aggressive management are needed for a
uccessful outcome. When any complication occurs, it is tempting to play
own its seriousness and hope for the best. However, a wait-and-see
pproach to perforation is likely to be lethal.

mergencies

Vho needs urgent endoscopy?

rue endoscopic emergencies (requiring immediate endoscopy) are quite
are. It usually takes several hours to assess and stabilize a patient with GI
leeding, or to evaluate foreign body ingestion by radiology. Whenever
ossible, endoscopy should be delayed until the bleeding patient has been
abilized hemodynamically. However, patients with persistent arterial or
ariceal bleeding may prove very difficult to stabilize. These patients
quire endoscopy for diagnosis and therapy despite hypotension. When
y patient with a known aortic aneurysm or aortic prosthetic graft
resents with acute GI bleeding, an aortoduodenal fistula should be
cluded by endoscopy at the earliest opportunity. Bleeding from these
stulae may stop for a few hours, providing a brief 'window' for diagnosis.
he second hemorrhage is usually fatal.

If a patient with acute dysphagia due to food impaction or foreign body
gestion is choking on secretions or has hypersalivation, complete esoph-
geal obstruction is likely. This constitutes a medical emergency. Foreign
ody retrieval and food bolus disimpaction is always safer when the airway
protected by a cuffed endotracheal tube. Most patients find endotracheal
tubation distressing unless they are deeply sedated or under a general
esthetic. The services of an anesthesiologist are invaluable in this
tuation.

ndoscopy in the intensive care unit

mergency endoscopy is often performed outside routine working hours in
e medical or surgical intensive care unit (ICU). Equipment is transported
om the endoscopy unit to the ICU on a custom-built cart which should
rry every instrument and accessory that may be required. Although ICU
atient areas have oxygen and suction outlets, tubing and connectors may

have to be provided. All aspects of emergency endoscopy take longer than you expect, so allow plenty of time. Endoscopists working in a large center may have the luxury of a trained endoscopy nurse or assistant 'on call' to help with the procedure. If, however, your assistants are unfamiliar with endoscopy, take the time to explain the procedure and their duties. The physician looking after the patient should be invited to watch. After the procedure, write a report in the chart. Do not forget to include post procedure orders. The patient's nurse should know who to call if problems arise. This information should be written in the notes with a telephone or pager number. Identify the physician responsible for the patient's care and communicate your findings and recommendations to that individual. As a gastroenterologist, you are likely to be the most experienced member of the team managing this GI emergency. If the patient is not directly under your care, you should be easily accessible for consultation.

Finally, the endoscope must be cleaned and disinfected after the procedure. Although we have come to rely increasingly on endoscope washing machines and automated disinfection, endoscopists should still know how to clean endoscopes by hand. At the very least, clean water should be sucked through the endoscope to clear solids from the instrument channel. If this is not done, the debris will dry and harden, requiring costly maintenance.

The acute GI bleeder

Endoscopy in the presence of active bleeding is a demanding procedure which should be performed by the most experienced endoscopist available. As the stomach and esophagus may be full of blood and clot, orogastric lavage using a wide bore tube is advisable prior to passing the endoscope. It is essential to protect the airway, as a sedated patient with copious blood in the upper GI tract is at significant risk from aspiration. An overtube will provide a degree of airway protection, but an endotracheal tube with the cuff inflated is best. Anesthesia and endotracheal intubation are essential for the agitated or combative patient. The anesthetized, intubated patient can be endoscoped in the supine position if necessary.

The endoscopist often finds a large amount of blood and clot in the esophagus and stomach despite orogastric lavage. Blood can be removed by suction but clots quickly block the suction channel. It is impossible to avoid every blood clot but if the instrument channel is kept clear by flushing (a water-filled syringe, or better still, a pressurized water jet, is a vital accessory) most of the blood can be removed. A large channel therapeutic endoscope should be used if available.

Blood and clot tend to pool in the dependent part of the gastric fundus during endoscopy. If this collection cannot be removed, rotate the patient 90°; this causes the pool of blood to move, revealing previously obscured areas. By patient washing and suctioning, the gastric mucosa can be cleaned and inspected. Regardless of the site of bleeding (whether it is in e esophagus, stomach or duodenum), a good view is essential for accurate diagnosis and effective endoscopic treatment.

A useful view is difficult or impossible to achieve when the volume of blood and clot exceed what can be removed through a lavage tube and the endoscope. If a patient has eaten within a few hours of the procedure, food debris will create an additional obstacle. When it becomes obvious that the odds against success are overwhelming the endoscopy should be aborted. It is remarkable how much better the endoscopic view can be just 12 or 24 hours later, once peristalsis has carried blood and clot beyond the duodenum. An incomplete endoscopy should not be regarded as a failed procedure: the experienced endoscopist will have learned something, even if the bleeding site is not identified. It may be possible to exclude certain causes of bleeding such as esophagitis, gastritis and varices, and the likely bleeding site localized, say, to the fundus of the stomach. This provides valuable information for the surgeon and interventional radiologist, should their services be required, and for the next endoscopist who examines the patient. If bleeding appears to be coming from the gastroesophageal junction or adjacent to it in the fundus of the stomach, the inflated gastric balloon of a tamponade device (e.g. Sengstaken–Blakemore tube) may provide effective hemostasis.

Endoscopy in the presence of active GI bleeding is a challenge: even experts have to admit defeat sometimes. Trainee endoscopists should take advantage of every opportunity to manage patients with acute GI bleeding, as expertise in this area requires considerable experience and technical skill. One must always be prepared to reassess the problem bleeder. It is sobering to reflect that despite the current sophistication of endoscopic diagnosis and treatment, the in-hospital mortality from acute GI bleeding remains around 10%. Aggressive resuscitation, careful observation and accurate endoscopic diagnosis are the basis for successful management.

The intubated patient

The use of endotracheal intubation to protect the airway has already been mentioned in relation to acute GI bleeding. General anesthesia and endotracheal intubation make endoscopy safer and easier in a number of situations. Although babies will happily swallow a pediatric endoscope, children from infancy to the mid-teens find endoscopy a frightening experience. Obviously, the decision to use anesthesia depends on the age and maturity of the child, but it is usually less traumatic for everyone concerned if a short-acting general anesthetic is given. Adults with mental retardation or psychiatric illness may also require general anesthesia. A few adults who become agitated under intravenous sedation or are frightened by their awareness during endoscopy may opt for general anesthesia.

It is essential to protect the airway when removing ingested foreign bodies, especially in children. Smooth, round objects easily slip out of snares and forceps as they are pulled through the upper esophageal

sphincter. If a coin or button battery 'escapes' in the hypopharynx, it ca
easily roll into the airway, with potentially catastrophic consequences.

Some endoscopic procedures are done in the operating room with th
patient already under general anesthesia. Immediate preoperative (
intraoperative endoscopy require some modification of standard tech
nique, as the patient is normally supine and cannot easily be moved. Th
first hurdle in the intubated patient is passing the endoscope. This
usually straightforward when done under direct vision. However, occa
sionally the upper esophageal sphincter cannot be identified with ease. It
often helpful to pass the endoscope using the blade of a laryngoscope as
guide. If you do not know how to use a laryngoscope, ask the anesthesic
logist to pass the endoscope for you, demonstrating its use. The inflate
cuff of an endotracheal tube can exert extrinsic pressure on the uppe
esophagus, causing resistance to passing the endoscope. This is remedie
simply by deflating the cuff just long enough to permit esophagea
intubation.

As the usual signs of patient discomfort are absent during anesthesia
take particular care to avoid excessive air insufflation during endoscopy.
a therapeutic procedure such as variceal sclerotherapy or laser photo
coagulation demands it, the patient's respiration can be suspended for
few seconds at a time to provide a stationary target.

Foreign bodies

Ingested foreign bodies are an infrequent problem for most endoscopists
However, every endoscopist should know the principles of foreign bod
management. Certain groups of patients are prone to swallow foreig
bodies, accidentally or intentionally; these include small children, th
mentally retarded, the psychologically disturbed (psychotic and suicidal'
prisoners and drug smugglers. The endoscopist usually hears about th
patient from an emergency room physician requesting help. A littl
detective work may render endoscopy unnecessary. First, it is sensible t
establish whether or not a foreign body was swallowed at all. The evidenc
is often circumstantial: a safety pin or coin may have disappeared in th
vicinity of a small child. Patients with ulterior motives, e.g. vagrant
looking for a bed for the night, may claim to have swallowed a dangerou
foreign body, such as a razor blade. Many such patients are repea
offenders who regularly swallow household objects, ranging from knive
and forks to paper clips and coins. Drug smugglers who swallow narcotic
sealed in condoms for transportation may come to grief when a packag
obstructs the intestine or ruptures, causing a drug overdose.

After taking a history from the patient and questioning witnesses, th
mouth and pharynx should be examined. In children, a small pin or pape
clip may have lodged in a tonsillar fossa. When adults claim to hav
swallowed a foreign body in a suicide attempt, look for burns on th
tongue, palate and posterior pharynx that suggest concurrent caustic o
acid ingestion.

Radiology is very useful for evaluating foreign bodies. A plain chest X-ray including the upper abdomen, and a lateral soft tissue X-ray of the neck, will identify the majority of radio-opaque foreign bodies lying between the hypopharynx and the stomach. In infants and small children, take plain X-rays from the base of the skull to the anus, as multiple objects may be present. Children frequently swallow coins, which are easily visualized on X-ray. Button batteries (the small ones in wrist-watches and hearing aids) should be recognizable by their 'step' profile. If difficulty is encountered defining or locating a foreign body on plain radiograms, a contrast study should be performed. Particular attention should be given to lateral projections of the pharynx and esophagus. Dilute (thin) barium is the preferred contrast medium. Contrast is especially helpful in localizing radiolucent objects such as plastics, fish bones and certain types of glass.

Not all foreign bodies need to be recovered. Indeed, up to 90% can be left to pass undisturbed through the GI tract; 10–20% will need to be removed endoscopically, and perhaps only 1% require surgery. Foreign bodies stuck in the esophagus or hypopharynx are of more immediate concern than those that have reached the stomach. Profuse salivation is a sign of esophageal obstruction that demands urgent attention. *Not all foreign bodies can be recovered safely use a flexible endoscope.* Ragged or irregular sharp objects, e.g. dental plates, may require the use of rigid esophago-scopy under general anesthesia. *It is essential to protect the airway at all times.* Young children will usually have their endoscopy under anesthesia but whenever there is a risk of foreign body aspiration, regardless of the age of the patient, the airway must be protected. Although an overtube provides a degree of protection during foreign body removal, the only way to insure airway patency is by the use of a cuffed endotracheal tube. Particular care is needed when retrieving coins and button batteries, which may dislodge from toothed forceps or a snare as they are pulled through the upper esophageal sphincter. When dealing with coins and other smooth, round objects, it is helpful to repeat a chest X-ray before endoscopy if more than 1 hour has elapsed since the original study: a coin or button battery may dislodge from the esophagus and pass into the stomach in that time, making endoscopic retrieval less urgent and some-times unnecessary.

Meat impaction almost always indicates some intrinsic abnormality of the esophagus, usually a benign peptic stricture or Schatzki's ring. Endo-scopy is necessary to define the lesion as well as to relieve the obstruction. Sometimes a piece of meat can be pushed into the stomach by gentle pressure using the tip of the endoscope. As it is futile to attempt to break up the material with biopsy forceps, a piece of meat that cannot be persuaded to move should be retrieved intact. Papain-based meat tender-izers are potentially harmful and should not be used. A meat bolus can be grasped with a standard snare or basket. The snare containing the food bolus should be pulled up against the tip of the endoscope as it is removed from the esophagus.

It is a good idea to prepare a foreign body retrieval kit or case. This should include a variety of snares and forceps: toothed (alligator) forceps are best for grasping coins and other smooth objects (Figure 2.19), whereas snares (Figure 2.20) and three-pronged graspers (Figure 2.21) may be needed for soft or irregularly-shaped items. The foreign body kit should also include an overtube (see Figure 2.6). Overtubes facilitate repeated intubation and provide a degree of airway protection. Rubber sleeves that fit on the tip of the endoscope can be used to protect the esophagus and pharnyx when removing sharp objects such as razor blades and open safety pins. When you need to retrieve an oddly-shaped object, it is helpful to perform a 'dry run' on the work bench using a duplicate item or a modeled approximation. This will indicate the most appropriate endoscopic accessory for grasping the object.

Which foreign bodies should be retrieved and which can safely be left to pass through the upper GI tract? As a rule, any object that gets stuck in the esophagus needs attention. This is particularly true of coins and buttons

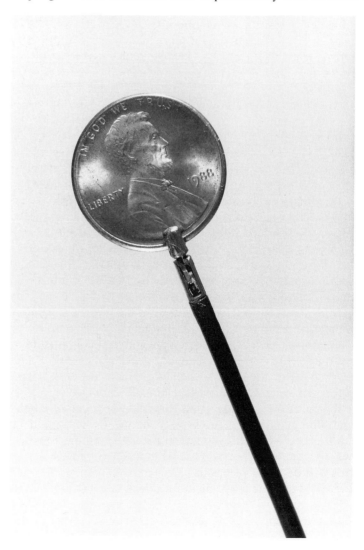

Figure 2.19 Coin held in toothed forceps

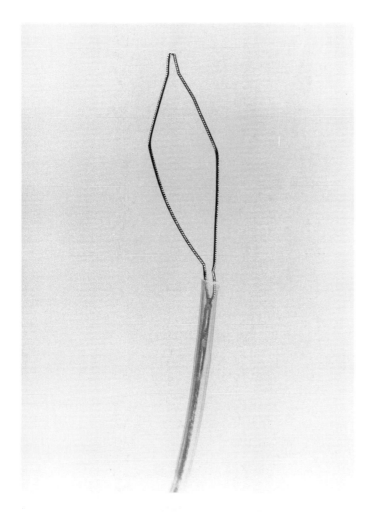

Figure 2.20 Endoscope snare

atteries: the former can set up an irritant chemical reaction and the latter elease highly corrosive contents. Once a radio-opaque foreign body has eached the stomach its progress can be followed by serial plain abdominal adiograms, provided that the patient remains well. For example, a coin an be followed through the GI tract by radiograms taken every 2–3 days. A sharp object (e.g. razor blade, open safety pin) that remains stuck in one osition for more than 2 or 3 days is likely to cause problems and should be ecovered surgically. Foreign bodies can also cause intestinal obstruction, articularly if they get stuck at the ileocecal valve. Safe passage of foreign odies is encouraged by a high fiber diet but cathartics should be avoided. Finally, it is wise to decline to endoscope patients for the purpose of ecovering plastic bags or condoms containing narcotics. Even if there are multiple layers of wrapping, these bags are easily ruptured, with fatal onsequences for the patient. The only safe way to remove them is by urgery.

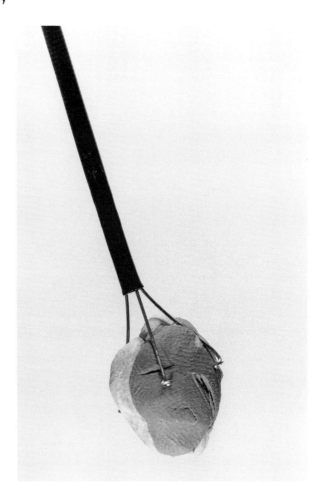

Figure 2.21 Foreign body held in three-pronged grasper

Corrosive ingestion

Corrosive substances (acids and alkalis (caustic)) may be swallowed accidentally (usually by children) or on purpose (as a suicide attempt). Fortunately, intentional ingestion of corrosives has diminished over the last 30 years following legislation controlling the availability and concentration of acids and alkalis available to the public. However, concentrated sodium hydroxide (lye) is still freely available in the form of liquid drain cleaner.

Patients who swallow corrosive agents may have chemical burns on the tongue, palate and posterior pharynx but their absence does not exclude esophageal and gastric injury. Endoscopy should be performed within 24 hours of corrosive ingestion to assess the extent of injury for management planning. A variety of scales have been suggested to grade injury, which ranges from mild erythema to gross necrosis. The risk of perforation at endoscopy is minimal if a flexible endoscope is used; rigid esophagoscopy should be avoided. The role of steroids in the management of corrosive injury is hotly debated. Steroid therapy should probably be avoided in cases of severe injury, due to the risk of perforation. Fortunately, extensive full-thickness injury requiring esophagectomy and/or gastric surgery is rare. Patients who have suffered corrosive injury to the upper GI tract are at risk of stricture formation and gastric outlet obstruction, and thus require close supervision. A late complication of corrosive injury is the development of esophageal carcinoma. As the latent period is unpredictable (may be many decades) no screening recommendations exist.

Basic therapeutics in the upper GI tract

Foreign body retrieval has already been discussed above. Although detailed technical discussion is beyond the scope of this book, the following basic therapeutic techniques will be described:

1. Control of hemorrhage
2. Dilatation of strictures
3. Percutaneous endoscopic gastrostomy.

Control of hemorrhage

There is no ideal method of endoscopic hemostasis. A large variety of techniques have been developed and many clinical trials have been performed, few with unequivocal results. Although endoscopists have felt for a long time that endoscopic hemostasis is beneficial, statistical proof has been slow to emerge. However, several studies have now been published that show benefit in terms of reducing transfusion requirements and the need for emergency surgery.

It may sound self-evident, but the bleeding site must be identified and clearly visible before any attempt at endoscopic therapy. A National Institutes of Health (NIH) Consensus Conference on the Management of GI Bleeding addressed the issue of which lesions should be treated endoscopically and with what therapeutic modality. Various stigmata have been identified in *bleeding ulcers* that appear to correlate with risk of rebleeding. Perhaps the best known is the so-called *visible vessel*, the bare end of a muscular artery. However, the base of a bleeding ulcer, or one that has bled and stopped, may be obscured by an adherent clot. Should the clot be removed to inspect the base? A firmly adherent clot on an ulcer that has stopped bleeding should not be pulled off. One overlying a bleeding ulcer may be gently lavaged; if this fails to dislodge the clot, additional force should not be used. Instead, endoscopic therapy (e.g. injection, heater probe) may be applied to the ulcer base around or through the clot. A non-bleeding ulcer that has no visible vessel or adherent clot has a relatively low risk of rebleeding and probably does not require endoscopic therapy.

The most common used treatments are:

1 Injection: with epinephrine (adrenaline), saline, sclerosants or alcohol.
2 Thermal: bipolar and multipolar electrodes; laser.
3 Banding (variceal ligator).

Less widely-available techniques include the use of clips and adhesives (e.g. cyanoacrylate), ferromagnetic hemostasis and the so-called endoscopic 'sewing machine'. New and as yet experimental technologies include microwave probes for thermal coagulation and the water-guided laser.

Injection therapy

Using a standard sclerotherapy needle (Figure 2.22), a variety of agents can be injected into and around bleeding vessels, including varices. In the author's opinion, sclerosants should be reserved for treating varices, as injecting them into an ulcer base carries appreciable risk of tissue necrosis and ulceration. A 1:10 000 solution of epinephrine may act by causing local vasoconstriction, although volume (and hence tissue pressure) may be more important. Some investigators have used 5 ml or more per injection without significant hemodynamic upset. Normal (0.9%) or hypertonic (1.8%) saline is an alternative to epinephrine, or the two may be combined.

Sclerotherapy of esophageal varices is most effective when the injection is directly intravariceal (Figure 2.23a). Paravariceal injection (Figure 2.23b) predisposes to ulceration and stricture formation and should be avoided. The sclerosants commonly used include sodium tetradecyl sulfate (STS), sodium morrhuate and ethanolamine oleate. To reduce local and systemic complications, the sclerotherapy needle should not exceed 5 mm in length, and treatments should be spaced at least 3 days apart. The total volume of sclerosant used at one session should not exceed 30 ml. To insure that the tip of the needle is inside the varix before injection, an X-ray contrast agent can be mixed with the sclerosant and the procedure monitored by fluoroscopy. An alternative technique is to connect the needle catheter to a pressure gauge and monitor intravariceal pressure.

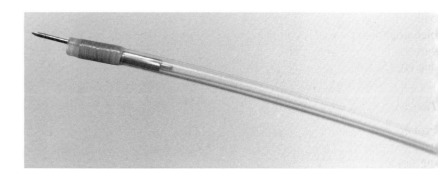

Figure 2.22 Sclerotherapy needle

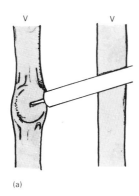 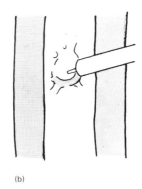

Figure 2.23 Variceal sclerotherapy. (a) Intravariceal injection (V, varix); (b) paravariceal injection

As most, but not all, blood flow in esophageal varices is upwards (cephalad), sclerosant should be injected close to the gastroesophageal junction. Usually 2–3 ml are used per injection. Until you are skilled at the procedure, the needle should be kept retracted in its sheath until you are ready to inject. Apply the tip of the sheath to the desired site then advance the needle. This is most easily achieved by having an assistant control the needle and inject the sclerosant. Terminology should be agreed upon in advance, e.g. 'needle in', 'needle out', and the assistant should report the ease or difficulty of each injection. Marked resistance is usually evidence of paravariceal (interstitial) injection. Both the endoscopist and the assistant should put on protective eye wear, as sclerosants are highly irritant to the cornea. The syringe used for sclerosant injection should point away from the operators and the patient at all times during sclerotherapy.

If a varix bleeds after the needle is withdrawn, advance the endoscope beyond the injection site and leave it there for a minute or two. This provides a degree of local tamponade. Persistent bleeding is an indication for repeat injection *below* the bleeding site. It is rare to have to insert a tamponade device (e.g. Sengstaken–Blakemore tube) to control bleeding after sclerotherapy. The success or failure of sclerotherapy depends on multiple factors, including injection technique, frequency of treatment, and severity of portal hypertension. Most endoscopists limit the number of treatment sessions. If esophageal varices have not been obliterated after five or six sessions, further sclerotherapy is unlikely to be effective. Gastric varices are usually unsuitable for sclerotherapy. As they occur within a few centimeters of the gastroesophageal junction, tamponade with the gastric balloon of a Sengstaken–Blakemore tube may be effective in acute bleeding. Gastric varices may appear following obliteration of esophageal varices by sclerotherapy; the definitive treatment is surgical decompression.

Thermal methods

Probes with *bipolar and multipolar electrodes* (BICAP, heater probe) are used to apply thermal energy to coagulate bleeding vessels and surrounding tissue. These probes have a conductive metal tip attached to a plastic

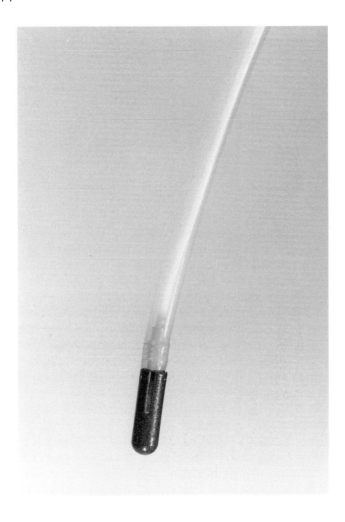

Figure 2.24 Tip of heater probe

insertion catheter (Figure 2.24). Larger probes are available for use with large channel therapeutic endoscopes. Current is provided through an electrical unit with a range of power settings. The insertion catheter has a central channel through which water can be pumped under pressure. This high velocity water jet is ideal for cleaning blood and clot from an ulcer base. The water also cools the tip of the probe. Animal and cadaver studies have shown that pressure as well as heat is necessary for effective coagulation of bleeding vessels. The combination of heat and pressure causes the opposing walls of the offending vessel to be welded, or coapted together (Figure 2.25). The usual technique for heater probe application is to coagulate a ring of tissue around the vessel before attacking it directly. Repeated application of the heater probe to one spot requires caution, as this may produce a transmural burn.

Laser (*l*ight *a*mplification by *s*timulated *e*mission of *r*adiation) is an elegant but expensive way to heat tissue. A variety of materials can be 'lased'; each produces light of a discrete wavelength with differing tissue

enetration and heating properties. The inert gas argon was the first source
f laser light with tissue penetration. Currently, the most widely used
ystem for GI work is the neodymium yttrium argon garnet (Nd-YAG)
aser. The laser energy is guided from its source to the target through a
pecial cannula or 'light guide'. The tip of the cannula is cooled by an inert
as, such as nitrogen, that is pumped through a central channel. As this
oolant gas, which is delivered at a rate of 2–6 liters per minute, can cause
apid distension of the GI tract, some arrangement has to be made for
xternal venting. A standard nasogastric tube, taped to the endoscope or
assed separately, is usually adequate. Laser has the advantage of allowing
reatment from a distance but is difficult to use with the endoscope tip
etroflexed, or in confined spaces. A new modification of this technology is
he water-guided laser. One of the drawbacks of conventional laser energy
s its tendency to cause such intense heating that tissue vaporizes rather
han coagulates. This can provoke bleeding if it 'punches' a hole in the wall
f the artery adjacent to a bleeding site. Using a water jet to 'carry' the
aser light to its target cools the tissue sufficiently to prevent vaporization.
his technology is still being evaluated.

The laser energy is usually delivered from a distance. Although contact
sers have been developed, they have not proved superior to existing
tand off' systems. After an 'aiming beam' is directed on to the target from
distance of a few centimeters, the laser is fired, delivering a brief pulse of
nergy.

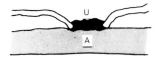
(a)

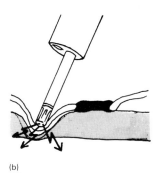
(b)

Figure 2.25 Coapting an arterial bleeding source using the heater probe. (a) The ulcer (U) has eroded into an artery (A) at its base. (b) Coaptation requires a combination of pressure and coagulation

anding

anding of esophageal varices is a relatively recent adaptation of a
ell-established treatment for hemorrhoids. Using a device that attaches to
he tip of the endoscope, varices are entrapped and banded. The rubber
and occludes the neck of the varix, which undergoes necrosis and sloughs.
his treatment is said to be technically easier, more reliably effective and
ess prone to complications than sclerotherapy. Data on the long-term
utcome of banding are awaited with interest.

Dilatation of strictures

he esophagus is the site of most strictures treated by endoscopists.
ertain strictures of the pylorus and stomach are amenable to endoscopic
herapy, as are a very few strictures of the colon and distal ileum. The
ollowing observations apply principally to esophageal strictures, but the
eneral principles apply elsewhere.

Esophageal strictures usually present with some form of swallowing
ifficulty, such as sticking (dysphagia), pain (odynophagia) or regurgita-
on of undigested food. There is considerable debate about the relative
erits of endoscopy and contrast studies in the evaluation of swallowing
roblems. A contrast study can yield information about structural abnor-
alities and motility disturbance that endoscopy will miss. However,

endoscopy offers the advantages of direct visualization of mucosa, th
ability to take biopsies and the opportunity for therapy. A contras
examination should be performed to assess tumors of the esophagus an
gastric cardia prior to endoscopic therapy or surgery. Contrast can als
define unusual anatomy (e.g. Zenker's diverticulum, tracheoesophage
fistula, webs, etc.) in cases of diagnostic difficulty. If a leak or perforatio
is suspected, a water-soluble contrast medium such as Gastrografin shoul
be used instead of barium.

When an esophageal stricture is diagnosed radiologically, the X-ra
appearances may indicate the likelihood of benign disease or malignancy
An exophytic mass causing obstruction is likely to be a cancer, but smoot
strictures are not necessarily benign. Endoscopic biopsies are required t
confirm a diagnosis of malignancy. This is particularly important in th
esophagus, where the histologic type (i.e. squamous cell versus adenocarci
noma) determines treatment options. It may be necessary to dilate
stricture before useful biopsies can be obtained. Repeated endoscopy fo
biopsy may be necessary to diagnose malignancy, especially when th
tumor is predominantly submucosal.

If an esophageal stricture will not easily admit the tip of the endoscope
some form of dilatation will be required. An endoscope must never be use
as a blunt dilator: this risks perforation. A newly diagnosed stricture tigh
enough to resist the passage of an endoscope should not be treated b
'blind' dilatation with mercury bougies. If a stricture has been diagnosed b
contrast study, or the patient is likely to have a stricture by history
endoscopy should be performed with fluoroscopy available. With th
endoscope at the top of the stricture, a floppy-tipped guidewire is advance
under fluoroscopic control. When the tip of the guidewire is well down int
the stomach, the endoscope is withdrawn over the wire. A variety o
dilators are available for use over a guidewire. Tapered plastic Savar
dilators are very popular (Figure 2.26) and less traumatic than metal olive
(Eder–Puestow, tridilator) (Figure 2.27a, b). These dilators come in sets
with external diameters ranging from a few millimeters to 17 mm or more
Sizes are often described in French (Charrière) gauge, a measure c
circumference ($\pi \times$ diameter (mm)). Multiplying the diameter by thre
gives a close approximation, e.g. an 11 mm diameter Savary dilator i
$11 \times 3 = 33$ French (Ch) gauge.

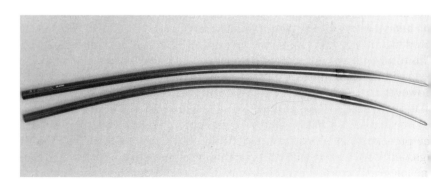

Figure 2.26 Savary dilators

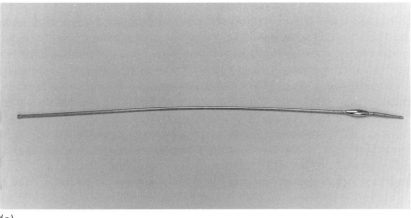

(a)

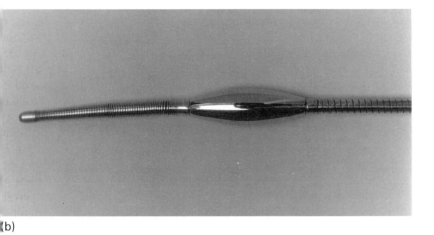

(b)

Figure 2.27 (a) Eder–
Puestow ('olive') dilator.
(b) The 'business end' of
the dilator

The rule in dilatation is to start small and increase slowly. Dilators
should never be forced against major resistance, as the impressive radial
and axial forces generated can result in a mucosal tear, bleeding or
perforation. It takes experience to know what force is appropriate and
what is excessive. Uniform resistance is expected and acceptable provided
that the dilator progresses smoothly through the stricture. Many endoscopists adhere to the rule of threes: from the time resistance is first encountered, no more than three dilators of increasing diameter should be passed.
This technique minimizes the risk of perforation. It is certainly tempting to
keep going if serial dilators can be passed, albeit with increasing resistance.
However, it is prudent to deal with a tight stricture by repeated cautious
dilatations over a series of days or weeks.

Great resistance followed by a sudden 'give' is ominous. If this happens
the procedure must be discontinued and the patient observed closely for
signs and symptoms of perforation. This may present as chest or back pain,
unexplained fever or pleural effusion or, more dramatically, with air in the

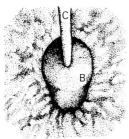

Figure 2.28 A through-the-'scope (TTS) balloon being used to dilate a stenotic pylorus. The cylindrical plastic balloon (B) is straddling the pylorus. The catheter (C), to which the balloon is attached (and through which air or contrast is injected to fill the balloon), is also visible here. This method of dilatation has the advantage of being under direct visual control by the endoscopist

subcutaneous tissues (surgical emphysema). The possibility of a perforation should be actively investigated by contrast study using a water-soluble medium. An esophageal perforation is a potentially life-threatening complication that should be managed in collaboration with a sympathetic surgeon.

An alternative to over-guidewire dilatation is the use of through-the-'scope (TTS) balloon dilators (Figure 2.28). These cylindrical balloons made of plastic are used under direct vision: you can watch the dilatation as it happens. Dilatations with TTS balloons can be monitored by fluoroscopy; as the stricture is dilated the 'waist' on the balloon disappears. To accentuate this effect, the balloons can be filled with a contrast medium instead of air.

Therapeutic dilatation of malignant strictures has very short-lived benefit. However, when a patient with an esophageal cancer cannot swallow secretions, even a transient increase in lumen size may provide a symptomatic relief until more definitive treatment can be instituted. Dilatation is often needed before an endoscope can be advanced through a malignant stricture. Insertion of an esophageal prosthesis is likely to fail unless the stricture can be dilated to the necessary diameter (about 15 mm for a standard prosthesis). Dilatation for malignant obstruction carries an increased risk of perforation because the esophageal wall is rigid; it is possible (literally) to split the esophagus.

Achalasia

Achalasia of the esophagus is a special type of 'stricture'. An aganglionic segment of the distal esophagus is unable to relax, causing functional obstruction at the level of the gastroesophageal junction. The esophagus proximal to the narrowing (at the level of the gastroesophageal junction) may dilate progressively over years and become extremely large. Achalasia is sometimes diagnosed on plain chest X-ray by the presence of a large gas shadow and air–fluid level in the posterior mediastinum. The diagnosis should always be confirmed by esophageal manometry before any attempt at therapy. Endoscopy is also essential, with particular attention to the gastroesophageal junction and a retroflexed view of the gastric cardia. A small tumor of the cardia may mimic achalasia: so-called pseudoachalasia. An achalasia-like paraneoplastic syndrome is a rare manifestation of certain extraintestinal malignancies (e.g. bronchus).

Dilatation of the aganglionic segment of the distal esophagus requires a dilator capable of exerting the high pressures (up to 300 mmHg) necessary to rupture circular smooth muscle. This is a high-risk procedure requiring appropriate training and experience. There is almost always bleeding after achalasia dilatation; after all, the aim is to disrupt the muscle wall of the esophagus. The risk of perforation is increased if the patient has had previous balloon dilatation, or achalasia surgery (Heller's myotomy). Patients who have had pneumatic dilatation for achalasia require close observation after the procedure.

Percutaneous endoscopic gastrostomy

Patients with stable, chronic neurologic disorders (e.g. stroke) who cannot swallow and those insufficiently alert or cooperative (e.g. dementia) to eat and drink may be referred for endoscopic gastrostomy tube placement. In selected cases, percutaneous endoscopic gastrostomy (PEG) is also an excellent way to decompress the GI tract proximal to malignant intestinal obstruction. The equipment required, including the gastrostomy tube itself, can be adapted from cannulae and catheters readily available in hospitals and clinics. However, PEG kits containing all the necessary materials in a sterile package are commercially available. The following are contraindications to PEG placement:

Peritonitis
Perforation of the GI tract
Stomach inaccesible for percutaneous puncture (e.g. following major gastric resection)
Presence of significant ascites
Abnormal stomach wall (e.g. malignant infiltration)
Irreversible coagulopathy
Tight esophageal stricture
Rapidly deteriorating medical condition.

An esophageal stricture is only a contraindication if it cannot be dilated enough to allow endoscopic access for the PEG procedure. There are several ways to perform the PEG procedure. A commonly used method will be described briefly. Although operating room sterility is unnecessary, attention to disinfection is appropriate, and an assistant is usually required. The patient lies supine with the left upper quadrant of the abdomen cleaned and draped, as for a surgical procedure. A complete EGD is performed before a suitable puncture site is identified in the stomach. This site must be free of any obvious blood vessels or pathology, such as an ulcer. The actual point of entry through the abdominal wall for gastrostomy tube placement is identified by transillumination and, occasionally, palpation with a gloved finger to locate the endoscope tip. Local pressure from the finger tip can be observed by the endoscopist as an indentation in the anterior stomach wall. Following local anesthesia to the skin and subcutaneous tissues, a small skin incision is made with a scalpel blade and an intravenous cannula is pushed through the abdominal wall into the stomach. A wire snare, advanced through the endoscope, is looped around the cannula, holding it in position. After the metal stylet is removed, a long silk suture is threaded through the cannula into the stomach (Figure 2.29). The snare loop is opened partially, slipped off the cannula and on to the suture, which is snared tightly. The snare is then used to pull the suture back with the endoscope out of the patient's mouth. The suture is tied to the gastrostomy tube, which is then pulled down into the stomach and through the abdominal wall with the help of external traction. After the gastrostomy tube emerges from the abdominal wall, the endoscope is passed again and the endoscopist coordinates the final positioning of the

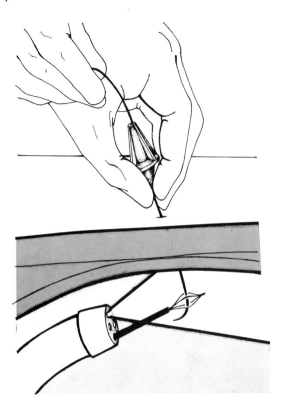

Figure 2.29 PEG procedure

tube with the assistant. It is common practice to give PEG patient
antibiotics to 'cover' this non-sterile procedure. Experience has shown tha
percutaneous gastrostomy tubes should not be used (e.g. for feeding, c
administration of drugs) for at least 24 hours after placement. Finally, it
important to be aware that a small volume of intraperitoneal air
frequently present for up to 1 week following a PEG procedure.

Bibliography

General

ASGE Publications, available from ASGE, Thirteen Elm Street, Manchester, M
01944

   Esophageal Dilation (printed May 1990)
   Gastrointestinal Tract (revised March 1986)
   Infection Control During Gastrointestinal Endoscopy (printed 1986)
   Role of Percutaneous Endoscopic Gastrostomy (printed January 1988)
   The Role of Endoscopy in the Management of Esophagitis (revised March 198
   *The Role of Endoscopy in the Management of Upper Gastrointestinal
      Hemorrhage* (revised March 1986)
   *The Role of Endoscopic Sclerotherapy in the Management of Variceal Bleedi
      (printed January 1988)

The Role of Endoscopy in the Surveillance of Premalignant Conditions of the Upper Gastrointestinal Tract (printed 1989)

vak, M. V. Jr. (1987) Technique of upper gastrointestinal endoscopy. In *Gastroenterologic Endoscopy* (ed. M. V. Sivak, Jr.), W. B. Saunders, Philadelphia, pp. 272–295

hitehead, R. (1973) *Mucosal Biopsy of the Gastrointestinal Tract*, W. B. Saunders, Philadelphia

austic ingestion

erguson, M. K., Migliore, M., Staszak, V. M. and Little, A. G. (1989) Early evaluation and therapy for caustic esophageal injury. *Journal of Surgery*, **157**, 116–120

ugawa, C. and Lucas, C. E. (1989) Caustic injury of the upper gastrointestinal tract in adults: a clinical and endoscopic study. *Surgery*, **106**, 802–807

oreign body removal

ebb, W. (1988) Management of foreign bodies of the upper gastrointestinal tract. *Gastroenterology*, **94**, 204–216

I bleeding

ilbert, D. A. and Silverstein, F. E. (1987) Endoscopy in gastrointestinal bleeding. In *Gastroenterologic Endoscopy* (ed. M. V. Sivak, Jr.), W. B. Saunders, Philadelphia, pp. 110–127

addock, G., Garden, O. J., McKee, R. F., Anderson, J. R. and Carter, D. C. (1989) Esophageal tamponade in the management of acute variceal hemorrhage. *Digestive Diseases and Sciences*, **34**, 913–918

ochhar, R., Goenka, M. K., Mehta, S. and Mehta, S. K. (1990) A comparative evaluation of sclerosants for esophageal varices: a prospective randomized controlled study. *Gastrointestinal Endoscopy*, **36**, 127–130

in, H. J., Lee, F. Y., Tsai, Y. T., Lee, S. D., Lee, C. H. and Kang, W. M. (1989) Therapeutic endoscopy for Dieulafoy's disease. *Journal of Clinical Gastroenterology*, **11**, 507–510

adonia, S., Traina, M., Montalbano, L. and D'Amico, G. (1990) Variceal ulceration following sclerotherapy: normal consequence or complication? *Gastrointestinal Endoscopy*, **36**, 76–77

IH Consensus Development Conferences (1989) Therapeutic endoscopy and bleeding ulcers. *JAMA*, **262**, 1369–1372

'Connor, K. W., Lehman, G., Yune, H., *et al.* (1989) Comparison of three non-surgical treatments for bleeding esophageal varices. *Gastroenterology* (1989) **96**, 899–906

anes, J., Forne, M., Bagena, F. and Viver, J. (1990) Endoscopic sclerosis in the treatment of bleeding peptic ulcers with a visible vessel. *American Journal of Gastroenterology*, **85**, 252–254

erblanche, J., Burroughs, A. K. and Hobbs, K. E. F. (1989) Controversies in the management of bleeding esophageal varices (in two parts). *New England Journal of Medicine*, **320**, 1393–1398; 1469–1475

Management of strictures

oyce, H. W. (1989) Peroral esophageal dilatation over a guidewire: fluoroscopy, endoscopy or 'blind' passage (editorial). *American Journal of Gastroenterology*, **84**, 358

Kozarek, R. A. (1987) Esophageal dilatation and prostheses. *Endoscopy Review*, **4**, 8–20

McClave, S. A., Wright, R. A. and Brady, P. G. (1990) Prospective randomize study of Maloney esophageal dilatation: blinded versus fluoroscopic guidance *Gastrointestinal Endoscopy*, 36, 272–275

Tytgat, G. N. J. (1989) Dilation therapy of benign esophageal stenoses. *Worl Journal of Surgery*, **13**, 142–148

Tytgat, G. N. J. (1990) Endoscopic therapy of esophageal cancer: possibilities an limitations. *Endoscopy*, **22**, 263–267

Vantrappen, G. and Hellemans, J. (1980) Treatment of achalasia and relate disorders. *Gastroenterology*, **79**, 144–154

Percutaneous gastrostomy

Ditesheim, J. A., Richards, W. and Sharp, K. (1989) Fatal and disastrou complications following percutaneous endoscopic gastrostomy. *American Sur geon*, **55**, 92–96

Klein, S., Hearne, B. R. and Soloway, R. D. (1990) The 'buried bumpe syndrome': a complication of percutaneous endoscopic gastrostomy. *America Journal of Gastroenterology*, **85**, 448–451

Ponsky, J. L. and Gauderer, M. W. L. (1989) Percutaneous endoscopic gastros tomy: indications, techniques and results. *World Journal of Surgery*, **13**, 165–17

3

Colonoscopy

Colonoscopy might seem to be simply an extension of flexible sigmoidoscopy but it is, in fact, a considerably more complex procedure. Flexible endoscopy of the rectum and distal sigmoid colon can be performed in most patients with minimal discomfort and negligible risk of complications. However, the difficulty, discomfort and risk increase as the endoscope is advanced proximally. For this reason, colonoscopy *cannot* be regarded as simply an extension of flexible sigmoidoscopy; it is a complex endoscopic procedure requiring supervised training and certification of competence. I chose not to include a separate chapter on flexible sigmoidoscopy, although beginners will find it helpful to gain experience in this technique before advancing to colonoscopy. For details of flexible sigmoidoscopy the reader is referred to one of several excellent textbooks on the subject. There is a long-standing debate about the relative merits of contrast radiology and colonoscopy. Each has its benefits and limitations. A barium enema is less expensive than colonoscopy and provides anatomical information unavailable to the endoscopist. However, the advantage of colonoscopy is that it offers a single procedure for both diagnosis and treatment. Contrast radiology and colonoscopy should be regarded as complementary investigations.

Indications

Diagnostic flexible sigmoidoscopy is generally indicated for:

1. Screening of symptomatic patients at risk for colon neoplasia.
2. Evaluation of suspected distal colonic disease when there is no indication for colonoscopy.
3. Evaluation of the colon in conjunction with barium enema X-rays.
4. Evaluation of anastomotic recurrence in rectosigmoid carcinoma.

Diagnostic flexible sigmoidoscopy is generally *not* indicated when diagnostic colonoscopy is indicated.

Diagnostic flexible sigmoidoscopy is generally contraindicated for:

1. Acute perforated viscus.
2. Severe acute diverticulitis.

Indications for therapeutic flexible sigmoidoscopy

All of the therapeutic procedures performed with colonoscopy may, under certain circumstances, be done with the flexible sigmoidoscope, provided that the patient is adequately prepared (e.g. polypectomy in the patient with subtotal colectomy, laser photocoagulation of a rectal carcinoma). However, colonoscopy, not flexible sigmoidoscopy, is generally indicated for therapeutic colonic procedures (e.g. excision of polyps).

Diagnostic colonoscopy is generally indicated for:

1 Evaluation of an abnormality on barium enema which is likely to be clinically significant, such as a filling defect or stricture.
2 Evaluation of unexplained gastrointestinal bleeding:
  (a) Hematochezia thought not to be from the rectum or a perianal source.
  (b) Melena of unknown origin.
  (c) Presence of fecal occult blood.
3 Unexplained iron deficiency anemia.
4 Surveillance of colonic neoplasia:
  (a) Examination to evaluate the entire colon for synchronous cancer or neoplastic polyps in a patient with a treatable cancer or neoplastic polyp.
  (b) Follow up in 1 year, then at 3–5 year intervals following resection of colorectal cancer or neoplastic polyp.
  (c) Patients with a strongly positive family history of colon cancer.
  (d) In patients with chronic ulcerative colitis: colonoscopy every 1–2 years with multiple biopsies for detection of cancer and dysplasia in patients with:
    (i) Pancolitis of greater than 7 years duration.
    (ii) Left-sided colitis of over 15 years duration (no surveillance needed for disease limited to rectosigmoid).
5 Chronic inflammatory bowel disease of the colon if more precise diagnosis or determination of the extent of activity of disease will influence immediate management.
6 Clinically significant diarrhea of unknown origin.
7 Intraoperative identification of the site of a lesion that cannot be detected by palpation or gross inspection at surgery (e.g. polypectomy site, location of a bleeding source).

Diagnostic colonoscopy is generally not indicated in:

1 Chronic, stable, irritable bowel syndrome or chronic abdominal pain; there are unusual exceptions in which colonoscopy may be done once to rule out organic disease, especially if the symptoms are unresponsive to therapy.
2 Acute limited diarrhea.
3 Metastatic adenocarcinoma of unknown primary site in the absence of colonic symptoms, when it will not influence management.
4 Routine follow-up of inflammatory bowel disease (except for cancer surveillance in chronic ulcerative colitis).
5 Routine examination of the colon in patients about to undergo elective abdominal surgery for non-colonic disease.
6 Upper GI bleeding, or melena with a demonstrated UGI source.
7 Bright-red rectal bleeding in a patient with a convincing anorectal source on sigmoidoscopy and no other symptoms suggestive of a more proximal bleeding source.

Colonoscopy is generally contraindicated in:

1 Fulminant colitis.
2 Possible perforated viscus.
3 Acute severe diverticulitis.

Therapeutic colonosocopy is generally indicated for:

1 Treatment of bleeding from such lesions as vascular anomalies, ulceration, neoplasia, and polypectomy site (e.g. electrocoagulation, heater probe, laser or injection sclerotherapy).
2 Foreign body removal.
3 Excision of colonic polyps.
4 Decompression of acute non-toxic megacolon.
5 Balloon dilatation of stenotic lesions (i.e. anastomotic strictures).
6 Palliative treatment of stenosing or bleeding neoplasms (e.g. laser, electrocoagulation).
7 Decompression of colonic volvulus.

Risks

As with all endoscopic procedures, the risks of colonoscopy are related to the skill and experience of the operator and the complexity of the case. The principal risks of colonoscopy are bleeding and perforation.

Bleeding is most commonly seen after colonoscopic polypectomy; it can be immediate or delayed. Delayed bleeding, which can occur up to 4 weeks after the procedure, is due to sloughing of the coagulum (scab) at the polypectomy site. Immediate bleeding usually results from transection of the polyp stalk before the tissue has been adequately coagulated (see below, Common abnormalities). Lower GI bleeding from a polypectomy or biopsy site usually stops spontaneously. However, if it does not, local methods of hemostasis (injection, heater probe) may solve the problem. Rarely, arterial embolization or surgery may be necessary to control hemorrhage. Routine coagulation screening is probably unnecessary but efforts should be made to correct known coagulopathy and reverse therapeutic anticoagulation. Drugs that interfere with platelet function, such as aspirin and non-steroidal anti-inflammatory agents (NSAIDs) should be discontinued 1 week before colonoscopy. If polypectomy is performed the drugs should not be restarted until 1 week after the procedure.

Perforation is the most serious of colonoscopic complications. Colonoscopy is contraindicated when the bowel is severely inflamed or when recent perforation is suspected. Pneumatic perforation due to excessive insufflation of the bowel proximal to a distal stricture is a rare event (Figure 3.1). However, this type of complication is an obvious risk in the presence of high-grade bowel obstruction. Forcing the colonoscope tip through a tight stricture also invites trouble. Perforation can occur in a normal colon. A colonoscope can exert enormous forces on the bowel wall. Sometimes these shearing forces are sufficient to cause a transmural tear,

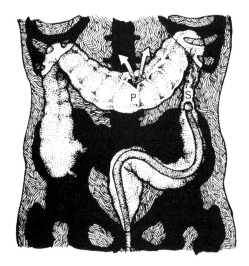

Figure 3.1 Pneumatic perforation of the colon. The site of perforation (P) is proximal to a stricture (S) that cannot be negotiated by the colonoscope

often at a distance from the colonoscope tip. A classic scenario is the sigmoid colon tear resulting from excessive force applied to overcome looping (Figure 3.2); this type of perforation almost always requires surgical repair. Balloon dilatation of colonic strictures carries a risk of perforation, as does electrocautery with a heater probe and photocoagulation with laser. The single most important factor determining the successful outcome of iatrogenic perforation of the colon is early recognition.

The postpolypectomy syndrome of abdominal pain, fever and leukocytosis without evidence of free perforation is the result of a transmural burn from electrocautery. This complication is almost always self-limiting. However, it is a wise precaution to put the patient on bowel rest and broad spectrum antibiotics.

Explosive combustion of colonic gases during electrocautery should no longer be a risk of colonoscopic polypectomy. Adequate bowel prepara-

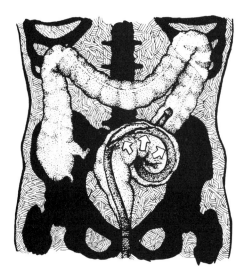

Figure 3.2 Linear tear (perforation) of the sigmoid colon caused by excessive force used to advance through a loop

tion deprives gas-forming bacteria of their substrates. Non-absorbable carbohydrate laxatives, such as lactulose, should *never* be used for colonoscopy preparation, as these are metabolized in the colon with the release of hydrogen and methane. As an extra protection against combustion, carbon dioxide (CO_2) insufflation has been recommended. As it is rapidly absorbed through the gut wall and excreted by the lungs, CO_2 causes much less bowel distension and discomfort than air.

Bowel preparation

As colonoscopy is usually an outpatient procedure, most patients prepare themselves at home. However, frail, elderly and retarded patients may require hospital admission for supervised bowel preparation. The extent of preparation required depends on the clinical indication: a patient with profuse diarrhea will require much less preparation than an elderly one with chronic constipation. Patients on oral anticoagulant therapy may require a brief period of hospitalization to withdraw coumadin (warfarin) prior to colonoscopy.

Standard bowel preparation for colonoscopy requires dietary restriction and purgation. Ideally, a no-residue or low-residue diet should be adhered to for 48 hours prior to the examination. As 48 hours is a long time to be on clear liquids only, 24 hours of a low-residue diet followed by 24 hours on clear liquids is a reasonable compromise. Flavored gelatine is a popular substitute for solid food but patients should be specifically instructed to avoid the red variety, which can produce what looks remarkably like bloody diarrhea. The optimum result of purgation is watery diarrhea, which indicates that solids have been eliminated from the bowel. Ideally, you should be able to read newspaper through the fluid the patient expels. Non-carbohydrate osmotic purgatives such as polyethylene glycol (Golytely) and magnesium citrate are now favored over castor oil and senna. It has been suggested that magnesium-containing purgatives should be avoided in patients with renal failure. Patients using these purgatives must drink plenty of clear fluids to obtain the desired effect. It is kinder to arrange for a timed purgation than to have patients up half the night before their examination. For a morning colonoscopy, purgation can be started around noon the previous day. The worst effects will be over by bedtime, and provided that the patient remains on clear fluids the bowel will stay clean.

If the patient is still passing any solid material by the time he or she comes for examination the preparation should be regarded as incomplete. It is useful to examine what the patient is passing in the toilet. If possible, a digital rectal examination should be performed before sedating the patient. A gloved finger covered with liquid or solid stool is evidence of inadequate preparation. Performing colonoscopy without adequate preparation is not only time consuming but unpleasant and potentially dangerous; the examination is prolonged because repeated washing and suction are needed to obtain an adequate view. At worst, the examination may have to be abandoned. Pathology is easily missed when stool is adherent to the mucosa. When preparation is inadequate there are several options. If staff and facilities allow, tap water enemas may be administered until the returns are clear. Often this is impossible in a busy endoscopy unit as a clinic room with a toilet and periodic assessment by a nurse are required. If the patient is from a hospital ward, he or she may return there for enemas. However, it is essential that the ward staff understand what is required. A small volume enema that is administered and evacuated within a short space of time is useless. At best, this will clear the rectum and the distal sigmoid colon. An adequate tap water enema requires at least 2 liters of fluid and this may have to be repeated several times. Standard bowel preparation is unsuitable for some patients, and others are unable to cooperate. For those who are intolerant of oral preparation, a nasogastric tube can be used to administer fluid and purgatives. There is also a variety of rapid preparation techniques that require patient cooperation and a comfortable toilet seat. As large fluid intake and losses may be hazardous to patients with congestive heart failure and renal insufficiency, these techniques must be used with caution. Obviously, they are contraindicated in the presence of known or suspected bowel obstruction.

Unprepared colonoscopy in active GI bleeding can be a miserable experience. Although blood is said to be an excellent purgative, don't count on it. Tap water enemas should be given or, if time permits, one of the rapid oral preparation methods employed. It is a legitimate concern that bowel preparation may obscure the bleeding site but most endoscopists are willing to take that risk. Less preparation than normal may be required when performing colonoscopy in the presence of active colitis, especially if the patient has profuse diarrhea. There is little evidence to support the widely quoted claim that colonoscopy preparation can precipitate or exacerbate a flare of colitis. Patients with a colostomy may have problems with bowel preparation; tap water enemas through the stoma can help. When patients with small bowel ileus or suspected high-grade obstruction (e.g. neoplasm, diverticular disease, Crohn's stricture) require colonoscopy, oral purgation should not be used. A disposable phosphate enema will provide rapid purgation and provide an indication of how much further preparation may be needed. Vigorous bowel preparation should be avoided in colonic pseudo-obstruction.

Colleagues who urge you to perform urgent colonoscopy in unprepared patients to assess bleeding or decompress colonic pseudo-obstruction might be less enthusiastic if they were the ones who had to do the procedure. With the possible exception of colonoscopy to decompress a volvulus, some hours spent preparing the bowel are a wise investment.

Which instrument?

To be sure of reaching the cecum, in the majority of cases a colonoscope at least 140 cm long is needed. For less extensive examinations, the 65 cm flexible sigmoidoscope is satisfactory; with good technique the splenic

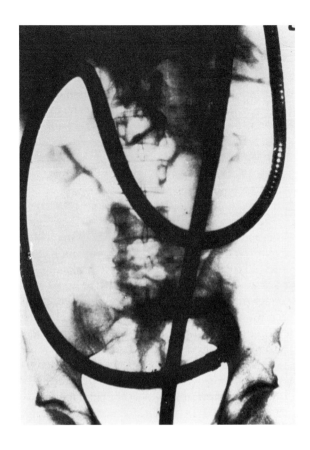

Figure 3.3 Colonoscope tip in cecum. Extensive loops can be reduced by straightening

flexure can be reached routinely. Although it is true that you can be in the cecum with only 65 cm of endoscope inserted, this does not mean that a flexible sigmoidoscope will get you there. Usually this 'short' position is achieved by withdrawing the endoscope with the flexible tip anchored; this maneuver is needed to straighten out the twists and turns (Figure 3.3). Video technology has greatly improved colonoscopy. The endoscopist is no longer glued to an eyepiece, sometimes in aesthetically unpleasant positions. Early video colonoscopes emitted a less intense light than their fiberoptic predecessors. This made it difficult to transilluminate the abdominal wall, an effect that can be useful for confirming that the cecum has been reached. However, subsequent generations of video colonoscope have addressed this problem. The choice of equipment is less important than becoming familiar with one particular colonoscope. For specialized indications, thin instruments (pediatric colonoscope) and colonoscopes with two instrument channels are available.

Sedation

As colonoscopy may be prolonged and uncomfortable, most procedures are performed with intravenous sedation. How much discomfort is felt depends on a variety of factors, including the patient's pain threshold and the endoscopist's skill. Compared with upper GI endoscopy, colonoscopy often requires greater sedation as, on average, the procedure take twice as long and is more uncomfortable. The same drugs are used as for other forms of endoscopy, but it may be necessary to 'top up' sedation during the procedure. Atropine and hyoscine derivatives used as antispasmodic agents or to dry up secretions are of dubious benefit and have unpleasant side-effects. The pulse oximeter is a valuable tool for monitoring sedation during prolonged procedures (see Chapter 1, Conscious sedation).

Colonoscopic anatomy

There is considerable variation in normal colonic anatomy. In addition, congenital malrotations may cause confusion. The full spectrum of anatomic variation is beyond the scope of this text. However, all endoscopists need to known the normal anatomy and common variants. It is useful to divide the colon into distinct sections as each has its own endoscopic characteristics (Figure 3.4). The *rectum* is recognized by its location adjacent to the anus, its ample lumen compared with other parts of the colon (short of the cecum), its semicircular valves and a characteristic mucosal translucency. The *anus* has always been difficult to evaluate at colonoscopy but, thanks to increasing flexibility of the endoscope bending section, the internal end of the anal canal can now be inspected using a retroflexion maneuver. It is important to become familar with the normal appearances of the anus so that normal veins and venous cushions are not mistaken for hemorrhoids or rectal varices.

The *sigmoid colon* loops anteriorly with the curve of the sacrum then posteriorly to join the descending colon, which lies retroperitoneally in the left paracolic gutter. The mobile sigmoid colon is one of the keys, perhaps *the* key, to successful colonoscopy. When the sigmoid colon is tethered in

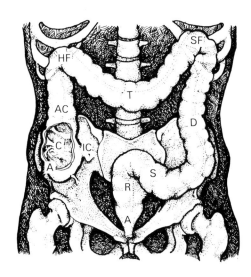

Figure 3.4 Colon anatomy. A, anus; R, rectum; S, sigmoid (pelvic) colon; D, descending colon; SF, splenic flexure; T, transverse colon; HF, hepatic flexure; AC, ascending colon; C, cecum; AP, appendix orifice; IC, ileocecal valve

one position by fibrosis resulting from previous surgery, pelvic sepsis (e.g. diverticulitis) or irradiation (e.g. for pelvic malignancy), colonoscope insertion becomes difficult and sometimes impossible. Excessive force applied to a rigid pelvic colon is painful and may cause perforation.

The *descending colon* is usually easy to negotiate as it runs a straight course up the left paracolic gutter before turning medially and anterior. Not infrequently a blue discoloration is seen at the splenic flexure where the spleen abuts the thin-walled colon. As splenic rupture causing hemo-peritoneum has been reported as a complication of colonoscopy, trauma to the splenic flexure should be avoided. The *transerve colon* runs adjacent to the anterior abdominal wall, then turns posteriorly to enter the hepatic flexure, which turns down into the right paracolic gutter. The *ascending colon* runs retroperitoneally down the right paracolic gutter to enter the *cecum*. The characteristic features of each part of the colon are described in the relevant section.

In summary, the colon is usually fixed at the rectum, descending colon and ascending colon. The mobility of the cecum is variable and depends on its posterior peritoneal attachment. The sigmoid colon and transverse colon are free to move on mesenteries. The mobility of these sections of colon is a function of the length and elasticity of their mesenteries. The splenic flexure has a false mesentery which allows some mobility. The mobility of the sigmoid and transverse colon mesenteries may allow loops to form; these are, in effect, iatrogenic volvuli. The sigmoid colon is the site of the so-called alpha loop (Figure 3.5) and, less frequently, the transverse colon may form a gamma loop, both named for the Greek letters they resemble (Figure 3.6).

The anatomic variations of the colon are numerous. Some are develop-mental anomalies, such as malrotation of the gut. Anatomic variations may be recognized if colonoscopy is performed under fluoroscopic control. The experienced colonoscopist rarely requires to use this, but during training fluoroscopy can be invaluable. If a barium enema has been performed

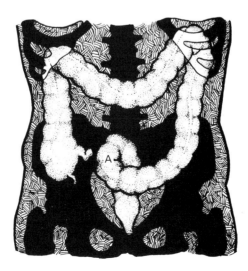

Figure 3.5 The so-called alpha loop (A) in the sigmoid colon. It is said to resemble the Greek letter alpha (α)

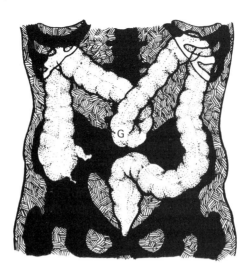

Figure 3.6 The so-called gamma loop (G) in the transverse colon. It is said to resemble the Greek letter gamma (γ)

prior to colonoscopy, the radiograms should be studied carefully for clues suggesting unusual or difficult anatomy. For example, a very redundant sigmoid colon (common in patients with chronic constipation) is a sure sign that the endoscopist has a difficult time ahead.

Colonoscopic technique: general principles

The expert colonoscopist has a feel for the instrument: sensing and interpreting resistance is as important as using visual cues to advance the endoscope through the colon. If the endoscopic view remains stationary as the instrument is inserted, this indicates that a loop has formed, often in the sigmoid colon. As the loop enlarges, the colonoscope tip may slip back as the insertion tube is advanced. When the endoscopic image suggests withdrawal during insertion, *paradoxical motion* is present. It is important to recognize this as further insertion of the instrument will only make matters worse. As a loop enlarges the patient becomes increasingly uncomfortable and agitated and there is risk of injury. The experienced endoscopist can recognize the subtle cues suggesting that a loop is starting to form: the loss of one-to-one correspondence of instrument insertion and image movement, a gradual increase in resistance to forward motion and signs of patient discomfort. Torque (twist) becomes progressively less effective as the loop enlarges. However, once the instrument has been straightened, torque can usefully be transmitted to the tip once more.

Perhaps the most common cause of failure to reach the cecum is over-insufflation. It is a frequent failing of novices to 'ride the air button'. Continuous air insufflation will maintain an endoscopic view but at the expense of grossly distending the bowel, which makes it more rigid. Distension is uncomfortable for the patient, who may become agitated and uncooperative. It is desirable to use a minimum of insufflation during insertion, relying instead on subtle visual cues to follow the direction of the umen. If you are unable to advance and there is no obvious loop, the colon may be distended and rigid. Try aspirating some of the air, withdrawing if necessary. If mucosa is sucked against the colonoscope tip during this maneuver, the suction can be released by uncapping the instrument channel. As mentioned previously, the use of CO_2 instead of air for insufflation reduces the risk of over-distension. If the air pump in your light source has high, medium and low settings, avoid continuous use at the high setting.

Positioning is very important. It is useful to change the position of the patient when it proves difficult to negotiate a flexure or to enter the cecum. Traditionally, patients begin colonoscopy lying in the left lateral position. Colostomy and ileostomy patients may be examined in the lateral position or supine. Abdominal wall muscle tone is one of the aids to inserting a colonoscope. In patients with poor or absent abdominal wall muscle tone (e.g. paraplegics) examination in the prone position may overcome this disadvantage (Figure 3.7). An elasticated binder can also provide artificial abdominal wall resistance.

Pressure on the abdominal wall at sites where the colon runs superficially can aid insertion. These sites are the left iliac fossa (sigmoid colon) and the left upper quadrant and epigastrium (transverse colon). Firm pressure is applied with one or both hands. As this is tiring, remember to tell your assistant as soon as he or she can stop applying pressure.

Stiffening the insertion tube can be helpful in difficult cases. Using a straight overtube, a twist or loop in the sigmoid colon can be straightened, allowing the colonoscope to advance further. However, in my experience inserting the overtube is often difficult for the endoscopist and uncomfortable for the patient.

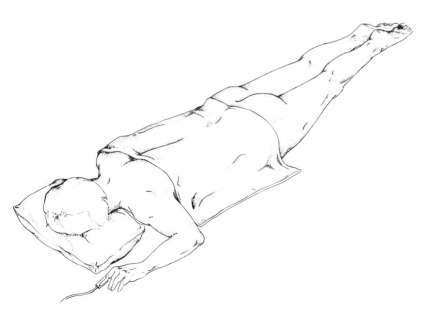

Figure 3.7 Patient lying in the prone position. This is especially useful for colonoscopy when the abdominal wall lacks muscle tone

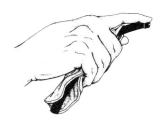

Figure 3.8 Hold 'scope with a damp cloth

Colonoscopic technique: getting started

Before starting the examination check that the colonoscope is working properly. Half way around the colon is a bad place to discover that the air pump is faulty. Make sure that the suction line is attached and switched on, and that air insufflation and lens washing are adequate. It is good practice to use a damp cloth to hold the insertion tube (Figure 3.8), otherwise you may transfer fecal material and secretions on to the control head. Aside from aesthetic considerations, using a cloth keeps the control knobs clean. Debris accumulating in the control mechanism will lead to more frequent maintenance 'down time'.

A brief digital rectal examination before starting serves a number of useful functions. First, it indicates how good or bad the preparation has been. Second, you may be forewarned of significant local pathology, such as large hemorrhoids, an anal fissure or a prostatic mass. Third, it mentally prepares the patient to have the instrument inserted. Fourth, it provides lubrication for tube insertion. Finally, it allows you to gauge anal sphincter tone. A patient with poor anal sphincter tone will find it difficult to retain insufflated air. Some endoscopists perform rigid anoscopy prior to flexible sigmoidoscopy and colonoscopy.

Explain to the patient that bearing down (as if to defecate) will make it easier to insert the colonoscope tip. The instrument tip should be inserted with lateral pressure and not end on (Figure 3.9). Insertion usually requires

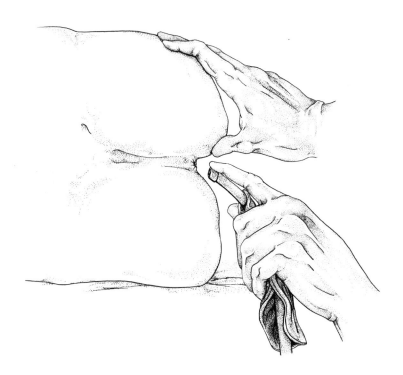

Figure 3.9 Insert tip with lateral pressure

wo hands: one to separate the buttocks and the other to hold the insertion
ube. It is helpful to have your assistant hold the control section. Do
lbricate the bending section of the colonoscope but avoid getting gel on
he optical system at the tip. There is a 'give' as the instrument passes
rough the internal anal sphincter. At this point, the colonoscope can
sually be advanced 5–10 cm into the rectum without resistance. A 'red
ut' is often the first view after insertion. When this occurs, the instrument
hould be withdraw a short distance and the rectum insufflated with air.
Vith the colonoscope tip seated in the rectum, you can take the control
ection back from your assistant and proceed with the examination.

Colonoscopic technique: anus and rectum

The internal end of the anal canal is best viewed by performing a
etroflexion maneuver. To accomplish this, the rectum must first be
istended with air. The colonoscope tip is then advanced along the
osterior rectal wall. Begin to retroflex before reaching the first rectal
alve. The actual retroflexion movement is achieved using full 'up'
eflection while continuing to push the instrument ahead gently (Figure
.10). To obtain the best view, some minor adjustment of the lateral
ontrols may be needed. Torque (twist) of up to 180° in each direction
ffords a circumferential view of the anus.

The rectum lacks the circular muscle rings characteristic of the descend-
ng, transverse and ascending colon. Instead, there are semicircular folds,
r valves, which are easily negotiated (Figure 3.11). Healthy rectal mucosa
as lustre and a translucency that allows submucosal vessels to be seen with
ase.

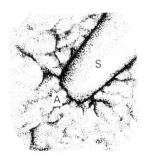

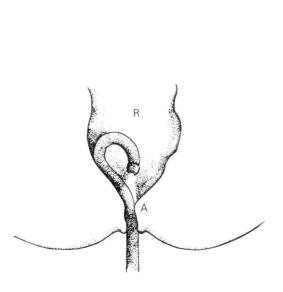

Figure 3.10 Retroflexion in the rectum (R). The endoscopic view shows the endoscope (S) emerging from the anal canal (A). The normal anus has a rather bluish appearance, due to vascular (venous) cushions that may be mistaken for hemorrhoids

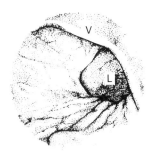

Figure 3.11 Rectal valve (V) with lumen (L) in the distance

Colonoscopic technique: sigmoid (pelvic) colon

The rectosigmoid junction is approximately 20 cm from the anus. This is the start of a number of bends. It is often difficult, if not impossible, to obtain a full end-on view of the lumen. Experienced endoscopists rely on other visual cues to guide them through the sigmoid colon. The sigmoid colon and distal descending colon are common sites of diverticula, which can cause confusion. The mouth of a diverticulum can look deceptively like bowel lumen. It is dangerous to drive the colonoscope tip into a diverticulum, as perforation may result. If the patient has had diverticulitis, the sigmoid colon may be tethered by adhesions. In some patients the sigmoid colon is so rigid that intubation is impossible. When there is major resistance to advancing the colonoscope and the patient is experiencing discomfort the procedure should be discontinued.

Patients often experience some discomfort as the sigmoid colon is negotiated. The degree of discomfort depends on a variety of factors, not least the skill of the operator. Local anatomic problems can add to the difficulty of the procedure. A loop forming in the sigmoid colon will cause discomfort. To straighten out this loop, advance the colonoscope into the distal descending colon, then pull back with the tip anchored. Until you perform this straightening maneuver the patient will be uncomfortable. Explanation and reassurance go a long way towards gaining patient cooperation; judge what the patient can tolerate and know when to withdraw or stop the procedure. The so-called alpha maneuver is a method of undoing a sigmoid loop; until the advent of increasingly flexible colonoscopes this maneuver was often performed under fluoroscopic guidance. However, fluoroscopy is rarely indicated now: it may identify the problem (a loop) but rarely provides the solution.

Colonoscopic technique: use of visual cues

If all that can be seen is a 'red out', the tip of the colonoscope is pressing against mucosa. Although insufflation can help when mucosal folds are lying over the colonoscope tip it is usually necessary to withdraw to regain a lumenal view. A 'white out' is an even stronger indication to withdraw: the pressure being exerted on the bowel wall is sufficient to blanch mucosal vessels. The patient may become agitated at this point, as pressure sufficient to cause a 'white out' is often painful. As in most situations during endoscopy when the lumenal view is lost, the correct response is to withdraw; resist the urge to push ahead.

Light and dark provide useful visual cues, light areas indicating proximity to mucosa, whereas the lumen is increasingly dark in the distance. Aiming for darker areas is one way to follow the lumen. However, this will not work if all you can see ahead are folds. The trick is to find where the folds converge (Figure 3.12), as this is usually where the lumen lies. The skilled endoscopist uses this technique to speed up the examination and to minimize patient discomfort. By following the lumen by fold convergence

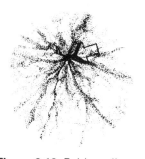

Figure 3.12 Folds radiate away from lumen (arrowed)

olonoscopy can be performed with greatly reduced insufflation. This
ake intubation to the cecum rapid as the bowel is minimally distended
nd therefore compliant. The colon is then distended as the colonoscope is
ithdrawn. As a better view is often obtained during the withdrawal phase
f the examination anyway, this is an entirely acceptable technique.

Another useful technique is to follow a path perpendicular to the
uscular folds. This will usually lead you to the lumen.

olonoscopic technique: descending colon and splenic flexure

he sigmoid–descending colon junction is commonly an acute angle. Once
is has been negotiated, often with a straightening maneuver, the route to
e splenic flexure is usually direct. The typical muscular rings (Figure
13) provide visual cues that help you negotiate the lumen. Advancing
rough the descending colon is often the easiest part of the examination.

The splenic flexure is normally a turn to the patient's right. However, in
out 5% of individuals there is so-called reversed splenic flexure due to
edial migration of the flexure on a false mesentery. The anomaly can
use difficulty in negotiating the transverse colon and hepatic flexure. A
raightening maneuver is required that involves counterclockwise rotation
f the instrument shaft. This converts the splenic flexure to a 'normal'
rientation, allowing the examination to proceed in the standard fashion.
o advance beyond the splenic flexure, it may be necessary to hook the
olonoscope tip around the angle and withdraw, thereby straightening it
Figure 3.14). The effect is sometimes dramatic; this straightening man-
uver may cause the colonoscope to advance rapidly across the transverse
olon.

Some endoscopists place great reliance on 'splenic blue' to determine
eir position. The spleen may be easily visible through the thin colon wall

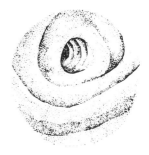

Figure 3.13 The muscular
rings and haustra of the
ascending and descending
colon

Figure 3.14 To correct a
loop in the distal colon, the
tip of the endoscope is
anchored (by angulation)
across the splenic flexure
and the insertion tube is
withdrawn, which
straightens the
colonoscope and removes
the loop. Some twist may
need to be applied during
this maneuver

(a)

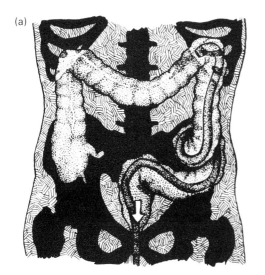

(b)

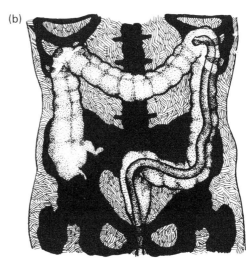

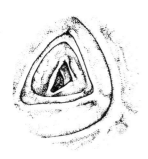

Figure 3.15 Triangular folds of transverse colon

at the splenic flexure, causing an oval area of blue discoloration. Howeve beware of over-interpretation; not all blue indicates the location of eith the spleen or the liver.

Colonoscopic technique: transverse colon

Advancing the colonoscope through the transverse colon is usually ur eventful. This section of the colon is recognized by its triangular folc (Figure 3.15). Difficulties arise when a deep bend or loop forms (se Figure 3.6). In both cases the solution is repeatedly to advance an withdraw the instrument, which straightens out the bowel. Pressure ove the splenic flexure or sigmoid colon may be helpful. However, when ther is a lot of redundant bowel it may be necessary to push cautiously throug the bends and loops before the endoscope can be straightened.

Colonoscopic technique: hepatic flexure and ascending colon

The hepatic flexure is recognized by some widening of the lumen, a bluis discoloration of the wall in the 12 o'clock position where the liver abut and by a turn 'downwards'. The hepatic flexure may be difficult to reach there is a large loop in the distal colon. Aspirating air to collapse bowe over the endoscope may help the instrument to advance. Occasionally asking the patient to take and hold a deep breath is effective. This flatten the diaphragm, causing the liver (and therefore the hepatic flexure) to b displaced downwards, which straightens the angle. Experiment with twis a little clockwise rotation of the shaft may be enough to direct the tip of th colonoscope around the flexure. The key to successfully negotiating th ascending colon from this point is aspirating air, as a considerable volum is required to distend the hepatic flexure. Once air is removed th colonoscope will often advance spontaneously as the tip drops dow towards the cecum. It has been noted that aspirating air lowers the positio of the hepatic flexure relative to the splenic flexure, which affords th endoscopist a mechanical advantage (Figure 3.16a, b). Obviously th disadvantage of aspirating is that you may lose the lumenal view. It is bes to repeatedly insufflate a small volume of air then aspirate, which allow you to see without grossly distending the bowel. It is often necessary t aspirate fluid from the ascending colon; the closer you are to the ileoceca valve, the most likely this becomes. If preparation has been suboptimal th cecum may contain liquid or semisolid stool. Apart from aesthetic conside rations, this is undesirable because dark material absorbs light, whic considerably degrades the endoscopic image. It is also easy to mis pathology when the mucosa is covered with stool.

It can be very difficult to decide whether or not you have reached th cecum. The appendix orifice (Figure 3.17) and the ileocecal valve are th

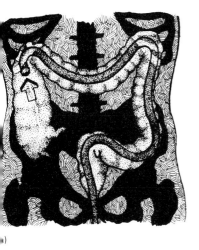 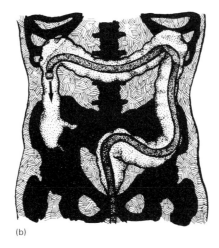

(b)

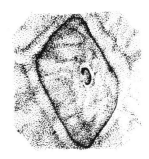

Figure 3.16 (a) To encourage the colonoscope to enter ascending colon, aspirate air. (b) The 'scope will often spontaneously advance when the ascending colon is decompressed. The tendency is encouraged by having the patient take a deep breath, which pushes the liver (and hence the hepatic flexure) downwards

most reliable landmarks (Figure 3.18). Transillumination of the abdominal wall in the right iliac fossa is a less reliable sign. Fluoroscopy may be helpful, but remember, the cecum is not always in the right iliac fossa.

Colonoscopic technique: ileocecal valve and distal ileum

The ileocecal valve lies 5–7 cm proximal to the base of the cecum. It is usually hidden within a rather bulbous fold, which may be more easily identified on withdrawing the colonoscope than on initial insertion. The colonoscope tip should be angled up and rotated until this fold is seen. The valve itself is rarely visible, although pooling of fluid may suggest its likely location. By withdrawing the colonoscope slowly with 'up' deflection and appropriate rotation the tip may lodge in the valve orifice (Figure 3.19). If you are fortunate, gentle insufflation is rewarded by a parting of folds and a view into the distal ileum. More often, however, the colonoscope tip falls out or slides off to one side. Patience is required to find the 'sweet spot'. Sometimes you can see through the valve but it resists advancement. If you hold this position for a few moments, normal peristalsis will open the valve transiently, allowing access for the colonoscope tip. The success rate for intubating the distal ileum increases with practice. If circumstances allow, ileocecal valve intubation should be attempted in every case, whether or not there is a specific indication. Gaining skill in this maneuver will be rewarded when you really need to inspect the distal ileum.

The distal ileum has a rather flat, lusterless mucosa when compared with the colon. In young people in particular there may be impressive nodularity, a cobblestone appearance, due to the presence of lymphoid follicles (Figure 3.20). Those who are unaware of this may mistake normal appearances for pathology such as Crohn's disease. With patience the

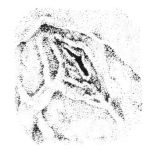

Figure 3.17 The endoscopic appearance of the appendix orifice

Figure 3.18 The endoscopic appearance of the ileocecal valve

Figure 3.19 To enter the ileocecal valve, the 'scope is advanced into the cecum and the tip partially retroflexed. The 'scope may then have to be withdrawn a little way to obtain the desired position

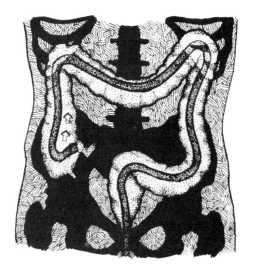

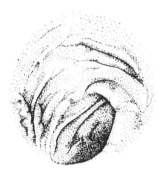

Figure 3.20 The endoscopic appearance of the distal ileum. A fine stippling effect may be seen, due to the presence of lymphoid follicles. This should not be confused with the more impressive 'cobblestone' appearance of ileal Crohn's disease

colonoscope may advance some distance into the distal ileum; this i encouraged by minimal use of insufflation, which allows bowel to 'tele scope' over the instrument.

Colonoscopic technique: withdrawing the colonoscope

As a whole, the colon is more easily and completely evaluated o withdrawal than on insertion. For this reason, care should be taken t perform a detailed examination on the way out. There is a tendency for th colonoscope to be expelled when forward pressure is released. This i encouraged by the untwisting of loops and the deflating of distende bowel. In short, unless the endoscopist exerts control over the withdrawa maneuver, the colonoscope may be rapidly ejected. It is impossible to loo for and identify pathology when mucosa is flying by at great speed Controlled withdrawal requires some tension on the insertion tube. Th patient may pass flatus during withdrawal, which collapses the bowe making inspection difficult. The bowel may have to be reinflated to allo adequate inspection. The colonoscope should be withdrawn slowly with rotatory motion of the tip. This can usually be achieved with twist an small up–down and lateral inputs as required to see behind folds. Th colonoscope tip should not be retroflexed intentionally except in th rectum and cecum. If you get stuck in the retroflexed position, do not pu back against increasing resistance. Instead, inflate the bowel, advanc gently (Figure 3.21a, b), then try again to straighten the tip.

When should you snare a polyp: on the way in, or on the way out? This i a matter of personal preference. There is a lot to be said for getting the jol over and done with when the polyp is easily visualized and the patient i cooperative. If you elect to leave a polyp encountered on the way in, yo may find the environment considerably more hostile by the time you ar ready to remove it, with fluid, peristalsis and patient agitation workin

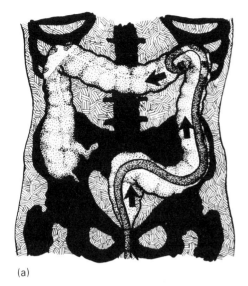 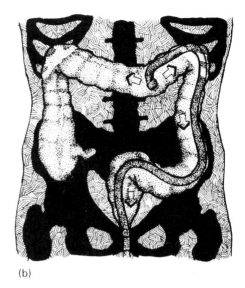

(a)   (b)

Figure 3.21 (a) The first stage of disimpacting the colonoscope is to advance, while insufflating air to distend the bowel.
(b) When the retroflexed tip is advanced into a wider part of the bowel, the tip can be straightend as the colonoscope is gently withdrawn

against you. Under normal circumstances, withdrawing the colonoscope or polyp retrieval then reinserting it should be a minor inconvenience. It is usually straightforward to pass the endoscope a second time as the bowel ill remain at least partially inflated. Colonoscopic polypectomy is dis-ssed below (Colonoscopic biopsy and polypectomy).

ommon abnormalities

large number of abnormalities may be seen during colonoscopy. These e well illustrated in endoscopy atlases. Some of the more common normalities will be described briefly.

olitis

he normal colonic mucosa has luster and translucency. In certain areas, rticularly the rectum, submucosal vessels are clearly visible. Loss of ese characteristics is an early sign of mucosal inflammation. Friability ase of bleeding) is another sign of colitis. The colonic epithelium is cked with mucus-secreting goblet cells; mucus secretion increases when e mucosa is irritated. This protective mechanism is responsible for the aracteristic mucous quality of colitic diarrhea. Severe inflammation nerates an inflammatory exudate giving the mucosa a mottled red and hite (strawberry and cream) appearance. Acute colitis may be focal or ffuse. Focal colitis is often limited to the rectum (proctitis), with a arply demarcated border between normal and abnormal mucosa. Most atients with ulcerative colitis have rectal involvement. Rectal sparing, atchy ('skip') lesions, aphthous ulcers, ileal strictures, perianal fissures and fistulae are all suggestive of Crohn's disease. As there is poor correlation between microscopic disease and macroscopic findings at colonoscopy, biopsies should be taken to exclude 'microscopic colitis' even if the mucosa appears normal. Biopsy at least two separate sites, one of them the rectum. Avoid taking multiple biopsies at a single site, especially when the colon is acutely inflamed: as the wall of the colon is thin, repeated biopsies may tunnel through to the peritoneum.

Infectious colitides tend to have non-specific appearances. However pseudomembranous colitis (associated with *Clostridium difficile* infection) is easily recognized: multiple cream-colored or yellow pseudomembranes dot the surface of the bowel. Cytomegalovirus (CMV) colitis may be suspected in immunosuppressed patients when large, flat, circumscribed red lesions are seen. These are different from, and should not be confused with, the nodular lesions of Kaposi's sarcoma complicating acquired immune deficiency syndrome (AIDS).

Ischemic colitis

Colonic ischemia is a microvascular phenomenon principally affecting so-called 'watershed' areas of arterial blood supply, such as where the superior and inferior mesenteric artery territories overlap. The classical presentation, usually in an elderly male, is of acute abdominal pain accompanied by a bloody stool. The diagnosis may be suspected from plain abdominal radiogram showing indentation or 'thumbprinting' of the colonic gas pattern: this is evidence of mucosal edema. As the condition is almost always self-limiting, endoscopy is only indicated if the diagnosis is seriously in doubt. The appearances of ischemic colon range from subtle to dramatic; at the severe end of the spectrum the mucosa has a dusky purplish hue. Once a diagnosis of colonic ischemia has been confirmed the colonoscope should be withdrawn. Attempting total colonoscopy may risk a mucosal tear or perforation. For the same reason (mucosal and mural friability) biopsies should not be taken.

Strictures

Benign colonic strictures may be postsurgical or due to a variety of conditions, including diverticular disease, Crohn's colitis, intestinal ischemia and tuberculosis. Contrast studies are often more useful for evaluating strictures than colonoscopy: the information provided by inspecting the lumen is often limited. It is unwise to push blindly through a tight colonic stricture, as this risks perforation. Some benign colonic strictures are amenable to endoscopic dilatation using balloon catheters. However, most require surgery. Malignant strictures may be obvious on barium enema examination. Colonoscopy is not required for biopsy of a malignant stricture if the patient is going to have a surgical resection, but an examination may be requested to exclude synchronous lesions, i.e. other umors coexisting in the bowel. Alternatively, colonoscopy may be performed about 3 months after surgery to look for polyps or tumors that have been missed. Frail, elderly patients with obstructing tumors are often poor surgical candidates. These patients may benefit from palliative laser ablation of the obstructing colon cancer. Circumferential application of Nd-YAG laser energy can enlarge a grossly narrowed lumen enough to relieve a subacutely obstructed colon. This treatment works best for low (rectal) lesions but here, as with every site around the colon, the use of laser carries the risk of perforation. Laser ablation of colonic tumors should be reserved for those patients who are unwilling or unable to have surgical resection or bypass. Occasionally, malignant colon strictures are extrinsic rather than intrinsic; locally metastatic tumor (e.g. gastric) encases the colon, causing narrowing but rarely complete obstruction (Figure 3.22).

Diverticula

These are outpouchings of mucosa at sites of weakness in the colon wall. They are easily recognized on barium enema. The presence of extensive diverticulosis on a contrast study should set off mental alarm bells: colonoscopy may be difficult! The sigmoid colon often becomes rigid as a result of the fibrous reaction to diverticulitis; this loss of mobility renders colonoscopy difficult to impossible. Other causes of a rigid pelvic colon include previous pelvic inflammatory disease, peritonitis, gynecologic surgery (especially abdominal hysterectomy) and pelvic irradiation. The colonoscope tip should *never* be pushed ahead blindly if diverticula are present. The trick to distinguishing the lumen (see Figure 3.12) from the

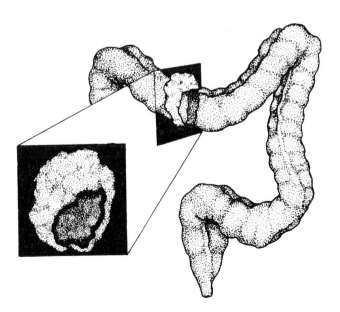

Figure 3.22 Encasement of the transverse colon by extrinsic (metastatic) tumor. Unlike intrinsic tumor (colon cancer), this rarely causes clinically significant mechanical obstruction

opening of a diverticulum is to follow the folds. Folds radiate from the lumen but not from a diverticulum.

Polyps and tumors

Colonic polyps come in all shapes and sizes. A major aim of colon cancer screening is the recognition and removal of premalignant polyps. Histologically, the important distinction is between hyperplastic and adenomatous polyps. Hyperplastic polyps are overgrowths of normal mucosa that have no malignant potential. They are usually small (5 mm or less) and sessile. Unfortunately, adenomatous polyps start off small and sessile too (microadenomas). These premalignant growths of adenomatous tissue may grow large enough to develop a stalk. Pedunculated polyps look not unlike mushrooms (Figure 3.23). The head may grow to several centimeters or more in diameter. Ultimately, some undergo malignant degeneration to form adenocarcinoma. As recent studies have shown that many small, sessile polyps are in fact microadenomas, even hyperplastic-looking polyps should be biopsied when seen at colonoscopy.

A positive histologic diagnosis of an adenomatous polyp mandates repeat colonoscopy every 2–3 years. When an adenomatous polyp is identified during flexible sigmoidoscopy the patient should return for full colonoscopy, as other polyps may be present. The adage 'once a polyp former, always a polyp former' holds true. If other polyps are not found at the time of the original examination (synchronous polyps), they may appear months or years later (metachronous polyps).

The likelihood of malignant change in a polyp increases with the size of its head, especially when the diameter exceeds 2 cm. If carcinoma is confined to the head of a pedunculated polyp (carcinoma *in situ*), polypectomy is curative. It is important for the pathologist to receive some of the stalk as well as the head. If the lymphatics of the stalk have been invaded by tumor, segmental colonic resection and a search for lymph node metastases is indicated. It has recently been reported that venous invasion of the polyp stalk seems to be less problematic. The technique of colonoscopic polypectomy is discussed below (Colonoscopic biopsy and polypectomy). Very large polyps may be difficult to remove at colonoscopy. Villous adenomas tend to have a broad base (they are often likened to a sea anemone) and can require surgical excision. Large sessile and pedunculated polyps may be removed in pieces; however, when these are clearly malignant, surgery is the appropriate management. Familial polyposis coli is an inherited (autosomal dominant) condition which carries a high risk of colon cancer. The definitive treatment is colectomy, not mulitiple polypectomies.

Most colon cancers develop from adenomatous polyps. These malignancies tend to present late in their course, with signs and symptoms such as occult blood in the stool (with or without iron deficiency anemia), altered bowel habit and unexplained weight loss. When the presenting symptom is bowel obstruction, the prognosis is particularly poor. Colon cancers may

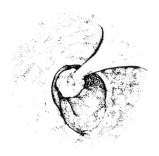

Figure 3.23 Pedunculated polyp

be polypoidal, annular or predominantly submucosal. Polypoidal tumors stick out into the lumen from one site (Figure 3.24), whereas annular (ring) lesions involve part or all of the circumference of the bowel wall (Figure 3.25). Submucosally-spreading tumors are difficult to detect. They are more easily identified by contrast study than by direct inspection, as they cause bowel wall rigidity. Submucosally-spreading tumor may be seen as a complication of chronic ulcerative colitis. As this type of tumor is particularly difficult to detect, presentation is usually late. Patients with pancolitis of greater than 8 years duration are at increased risk of colon cancer. Colonoscopic surveillance in ulcerative colitis requires multiple biopsies to look for dysplasia, a premalignant change. When serial biopsies show progressively worsening dysplasia, or severe dysplasia is present on one or two occasions, total colectomy is usually recommended. Connective tissue tumors of the colon are rare. Tumor metastasis to the colon is usually by direct spread from adjacent organs such as stomach, uterine cervix, bladder and prostate. In AIDS patients, Kaposi's sarcoma may affect the GI tract, causing the mucosa to be studded with small, slightly raised, purplish lesions.

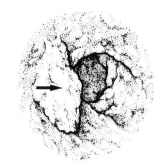

Figure 3.24 Polypoidal tumor (arrowed), protruding into lumen of the colon

Telangiectasia

These are vascular malformations akin to so-called spider naevi on the skin. They are dilated arterioles with surfaces branching that form rose-colored spots on the mucosal surface. Telangiectasia are friable and may bleed actively enough to cause overt rectal bleeding. More often, however, they are discovered during a search for the cause of chronic anemia or occult blood in the stool. Telangiectasia can occur anywhere in the GI tract, and may be familial (as in the Osler–Rendu–Weber syndrome) or acquired. The latter are particularly associated with chronic renal failure and aortic valve stenosis. Endoscopic ablation may be effective for solitary lesions, but surgery (segmental resection) should be considered if a large number are found in one location. Frequently, however, telangiectasia are too diffuse for surgical management. Hormonal therapy (with estrogens) has been used with reported benefit in such patients.

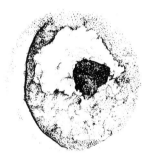

Figure 3.25 Annular tumor

Colonoscopic biopsy and polypectomy

Biopsy

Biopsy technique in the colon is similar to that used elsewhere in the bowel. However, colonic biopsy forceps have to travel a considerable distance to reach their target. When the bending section of the colonoscope is flexed, biopsy forceps may refuse to advance through the tip. When this happens, the colonoscope should be withdrawn a short distance and the tip straightened as much as possible, consistent with maintaining reasonable position in the bowel. It may be necessary to pull back from the

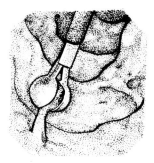

Figure 3.26 Hot biopsy forceps. Mucosa has been pulled up to create a pseudostalk

intended biopsy site, pass the forceps until they appear at the colonoscope tip, then advance, taking care not to traumatize the bowel wall. Fluoroscopy may occasionally help to identify the cause of mechanical resistance.

Hot biopsy is a useful technique that destroys small polyps as you biopsy them. Using standard biopsy forceps with insulation, current can be applied from an electrocautery unit. The tip of the polyp is grasped by the forceps and pulled into the lumen (Figure 3.26). A brief application of coagulating current burns off the mucosal 'stalk' created by traction. However, the current does not damage the tissue inside the forceps, which is retrieved as a standard biopsy specimen.

Polypectomy

Colonoscopic polypectomy can be a very simple procedure, or one requiring considerable skill, depending on the circumstances. An understanding of the principles of electrocautery is essential. A wire snare is used to entrap the polyp base or stalk, through which current is applied. Snares come in all shapes and sizes. Basically a snare is a long loop of wire covered with an insulating plastic sheath (Figure 3.27). Movements of the

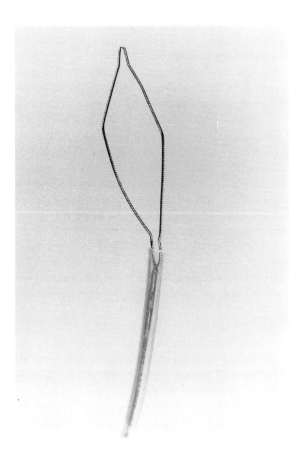

Figure 3.27 Polypectomy snare

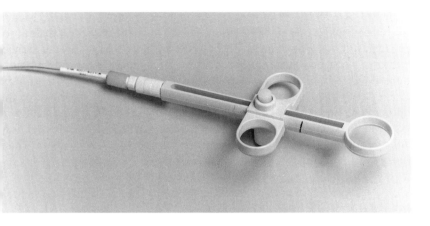

Figure 3.28 Polypectomy snare handle marked to indicate where snare fully retracted (1–2 cm) within its plastic sheath

andle control opening and closing of the wire loop. Before passing a
1are, it should be inspected and marked. Using a pencil or marker, draw a
ne across the handle to indicate the position at which the wire loop is just
ithin its sheath (Figure 3.28). This indicates when the stalk of the polyp is
ear to being transected, which should only be attempted after adequate
oagulation. At the fully closed position, the wire loop should be retracted
–2 cm within the sheath (Figure 3.29). If it is not, you may be unable to
ansect the polyp stalk once it has been coagulated.

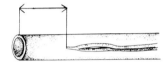

Figure 3.29 Optimal position for polypectomy snare wire when handle in fully closed position: 1–2 cm inside plastic sheath

If a polyp is sessile, a pseudostalk can be created by snaring the base and
fting it away from the surrounding mucosa (Figure 3.30). Pedunculated
olyps are snared over the head; the loop is then positioned for cutting
round the stalk (Figure 3.31). It often seems that polyps assume the worst
ossible orientation for snaring: they hide behind folds or have such long
talks that the head is hidden around the next bend (Figure 3.32). Even if a
olyp is easily visualized, the snare may come out of the instrument
hannel at 90° to the desired orientation. Patience is required, as well as a
ooperative patient. You cannot safely snare polyps and use electrocautery
hen the bowel is in constant motion due to peristalsis or patient agitation.
f the patient is unable to retain insufflated air, the procedure will be
onsiderably more difficult. You should take a few moments to assess
edation before proceeding with polypectomy. There is often a 'natural
reak' in the procedure as a grounding plate is applied and the electrocaut-
ry circuit checked; this is a good time to evaluate the patient and 'top up'
edation if required.

To grasp the polyp, open the snare fully and maneuver the loop over the
ead. Avoid opening the snare rapidly, as this can damage or even
erforate the bowel wall. Exact positioning requires delicate movements of
1e colonoscope controls and some back and forward movement of the
haft. Try to place the end of the insulating sheath against the stalk near
but not at) its base and slowly tighten the snare (Figure 3.33). This will
1aintain your position. If you drag the snare back over the polyp, the wire
oop may skim over the top (Figure 3.34). *Do not close the loop fully* (i.e.

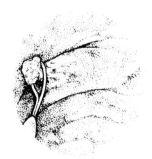

Figure 3.30 Using a snare to remove a small polyp. Traction can be used to create a short pseudostalk

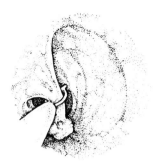

Figure 3.31 Good position for polypectomy. The snare is far enough down the stalk to leave a useful margin for the pathologist, while being far enough from the base of the stalk to avoid causing a mural burn

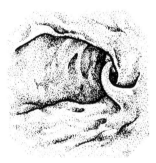

Figure 3.32 Polyp head hidden behind fold

to the mark you made on the handle): if you transect the stalk withou adequate cautery, bleeding is likely.

When removing a sessile polyp by snare cautery, tension must be applie to lift the polyp away from the bowel wall. Leave part of the wire loop fre behind the stalk of a pedunculated polyp. This reduces the amount of wir in contact with tissue, which increases current density. If the polyp canno be snared by lowering the loop over the head, a 'reverse looping' maneuve may solve the problem: the tip of the snare is positioned at the base of th polyp, then the snare is opened. This forces the loop backwards over th polyp, which can then be snared. Do not snare the stalk right against th mucosa, as this risks thermal injury (a transmural burn) to the bowel. A the other extreme, do not snare the stalk at the level of the head, as thi will leave no stalk for the pathologist.

Start the polypectomy with short bursts of coagulating current alone You should see evidence of coagulation (blanching in the vicinity of th wire) within seconds. Tightening the loop causes a rapid increase i heating. Very rapid heating should be avoided; enough time should elaps to ensure coagulation of blood vessels in the stalk. If no coagulation i observed, the wire loop should be tightened a little to increase curren density, but avoid transecting the stalk. If this fails, increase the setting o the electrocautery control by one or two increments. If there is still n visible effect, stop and carefully check all the electrical connections. A break in the grounding wire may be invisible so try using a different one Finally, try repositioning the snare, which may have caught part of th head as well as the stalk (Figure 3.35). The result of snare malposition i that the current has to heat a much greater volume of tissue than you think with apparent lack of effect. Finally, if the head of the polyp is touchin bowel wall some energy may be dissipated by 'heat sink' effect (Figur 3.36). In practice, this is rarely a significant problem.

Excessive coagulation without cutting should be avoided for two rea sons. First, the heat generated will eventually be transmitted to the bowe wall. Second, if the stalk is excessively desiccated by 'slow cooking', cuttin becomes difficult. The wire may become embedded in the stalk, especiall if it is tightened in an effort to accelerate the cut. At this point it may prov difficult to release the polyp from the snare. Tightening the snare beyon

Figure 3.33 Polypectomy. Advance the sleeve of the snare until it touches the stalk of the polyp. The wire is then slowly tightened until it is loosely around the stalk. Great care must be taken to avoid accidental transection of the stalk before electrocautery can be applied

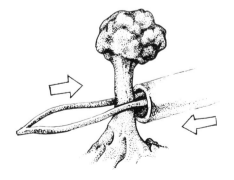

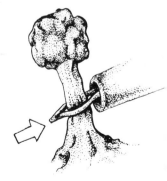

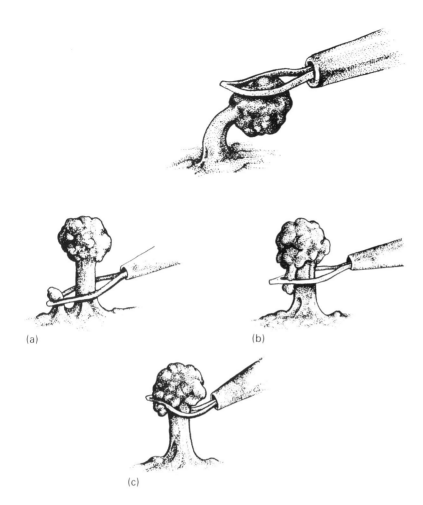

(a)

(b)

(c)

Figure 3.34 The snare may skim over the head of the polyp

Figure 3.35 Three technical problems that render polypectomy more difficult. (a) A fold of normal mucosa has been caught as the snare is tightened around the stalk. Due to extension of tissue from the polyp head (b), or malposition of the snare (c), the snare may have to cut through neoplastic tissue as well as stalk. Each situation increases the amount of electrocautery required, making the cut slower and less efficient. Problem (a) also risks perforation or transmural burn through normal colon

he full closure mark should transect the stalk (which explains why checking and marking the snare *before* you attempt polypectomy is so important). Rarely, a brief burst of cutting current is needed to complete the job.

Very large polyps may resist standard snare resection. If the polyp head is too large or irregular to snare completely, it can be removed in pieces. Large stalks are a problem. The larger the stalk, the more likely it is to contain large blood vessels. As external heating can be insufficient to coagulate the core, the stump may bleed profusely after polypectomy. One way to deal with this problem is to use a double channel colonoscope to pass two snares, one above the other. The snare nearer the polyp head is used to perform the polypectomy. If the stump then starts to bleed, the lower snare is tightened and coagulating current applied for hemostasis. An alternative approach is to inject the stalk with several milliliters of 1:10 000 epinephrine solution prior to polypectomy. The local ischemia produced may reduce the risk of immediate postpolypectomy bleeding. However, it does not prevent delayed hemorrhage.

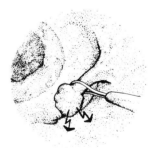

Figure 3.36 Heat sink effect. If the head of the polyp is in contact with bowel wall, current can be dissipated, reducing the effectiveness of polypectomy. The risk of a burn to the wall in contact with the polyp head is more theoretical than real

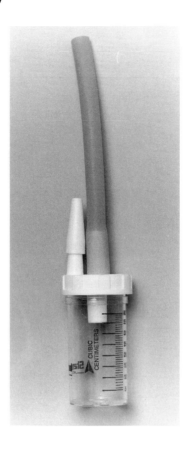

Figure 3.37 Suction trap

The polyp should be recovered for histologic examination. Small polyp can be sucked through the colonoscope into a specimen trap, a plasti container placed in the suction path to collect material (Figure 3.37) Larger polyps may be sucked on to the tip of the colonoscope, which i then withdrawn. However, not infrequently the polyp is dislodged when i meets resistance at the internal anal sphincter. Polyps lying free in th rectum can often be removed with a gloved finger. A secure way to recove polyps is to grasp them with a snare, basket or purpose-built three-pronge grabber (Figure 3.38). Once the transected polyp has been secured, i should be pulled firmly against the colonoscope tip before the instrument i withdrawn. As resected polyps undergo rapid autolysis (tissue breakdown the specimen should be placed immediately in formalin. If a polyp canno be recovered endoscopically (sometimes they tumble off into the distance a tap-water enema administered at the end of the procedure will help. Th polyp is usually in the return, which should be collected and sieved.

Polypectomy is the most common therapeutic maneuver performe during colonoscopy. However, there are endoscopic means of hemostasis tumor ablation, stricture dilatation and colonic decompression. It i beyond the scope of this book to describe these in detail. However techniques for decompression of sigmoid volvuli and pseudo-obstructio will be mentioned briefly.

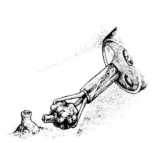

Figure 3.38 The polyp head is recovered using a three-pronged grasping device

Decompression techniques

Volvuli are twists in the bowel. Parts of the colon with mesentery are susceptible to twisting around on themselves, causing mechanical obstruction. The most common type is the sigmoid volvulus (Figure 3.39). Volvuli may spontaneously unwind and decompress, but often assistance is required. The definitive treatment is surgical: the twist is undone and a '-pexy' procedure performed to anchor the offending segment of bowel in place. This is recommended for recurrent volvuli. However, in the acute situation it is worth trying to decompress a volvulus without recourse to surgery. An experienced radiologist may do this during the course of a contrast study by carefully advancing a rubber tube through the 'neck' of the volvulus. Successful decompression results in an explosive rush of barium. Similarly, by gentle probing, the tip of a colonoscope or flexible sigmoidoscope can be advanced into the spiral lumen of the volvulus. The instrument is advanced and rotated (usually counterclockwise) to untwist the bowel.

Pseudo-obstruction (Ogilvie's syndrome) is the term given to a non-obstructive ileus of the large intestine. It is usually seen in debilitated patients in the ICU who may have severe infection and/or metabolic upset. Narcotic analgesics and phenothiazines (e.g. antiemetics) are contributory

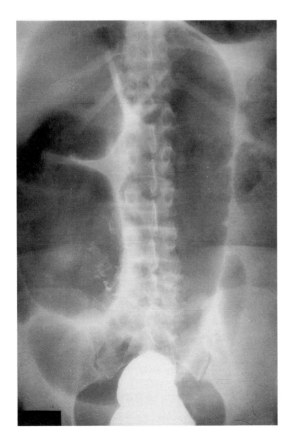

Figure 3.39 Sigmoid volvulus

factors. The smooth muscle of the colon loses tone, resulting in colon dilatation. There is good evidence that rapid dilatation of the colon, or persistent dilatation of the cecum to a diameter of greater than 12 cm for 48 hours or more, is associated with risk of perforation and peritonitis. Although the definitive treatment of pseudo-obstruction is that of the primary cause, the endoscopist may be asked to decompress the colon. As the problem is loss of tone, colonoscopy to the cecum with aspiration of air during withdrawal is a waste of time. Not only is this an unpleasant procedure (the bowel is usually unprepared) but the colon distends in front of your eyes as the colonoscope is withdrawn. Colonoscopy is only useful in pseudo-obstruction if a decompression tube is left for continuous aspiration. The standard technique is to advance the decompression tube through the instrument channel as the colonoscope is withdrawn. This can be monitored by fluoroscopy if the tube has a guidewire of central stylet. The decompression tube should be connected to low, intermittent wall suction. There is considerable debate about the effectiveness of endoscopic decompression of the colon. However, when it works the effect is gratifying (and sometimes spectacular).

Bibliography

General

ASGE Publications, available from ASGE, Thirteen Elm Street, Manchester, MA 01944:

> *Flexible Sigmoidoscopy* (revised March 1986)
> *The Role of Colonoscopy in the Management of Patients with Colonic Polyps* (revised May 1986)
> *The Role of Colonoscopy in the Management of Patients with Inflammatory Bowel Disease* (revised May 1986)
> *The Role of Endoscopy in the Patient with Lower Gastrointestinal Bleeding* (printed May 1986)

Connolly, G. M., Forbes, A., Gleeson, J. A. and Gazzard, B. G. (1990) The value of barium enema and colonoscopy in patients infected with HIV. *AIDS*, **4**, 687–689

Rex, D., Weddle, R., Lehman, G. *et al* (1990) Air contrast barium enema *versus* colonoscopy for suspected lower gastrointestinal bleeding. *Gastroenterology*, **98**, 855–861

Rogers, B. H. (1990) Colonoscopy with fluoroscopy (editorial). *Gastrointestinal Endoscopy*, **36**, 71–72

Sakai, Y. (1987) Technique of colonoscopy. In *Gastroenterologic Endoscopy* (ed. M. V. Sivak, Jr), W. B. Saunders, Philadelphia, pp. 840–867

Surawicz, C. M. (1987) Diagnosing colitis. Biopsy is best. *Gastroenterology*, **92**, 538–540

Waye, J. D. (1990) Colonoscopy without fluoroscopy (editorial). *Gastrointestinal Endoscopy*, **36**, 72–73

Waye, J. D. and Bashkoff, E. (1991) Total colonoscopy: is it always possible? *Gastrointestinal Endoscopy*, **37**, 152–154

Waye, J. D., Yessayan, S. A., Lewis, B. S. and Fabry, T. L. (1990) The technique of abdominal pressure in total colonoscopy. *Gastrointestinal Endoscopy*, **37**, 147–151

Williams, C. B. and Bedenne, L. (1990) Management of colorectal polyps: is all the effort worthwhile? *Journal of Gastroenterology and Hepatology*, **5**, 144–165

Bowel preparation

Jonas, G., Mahoney, A., Murray, J. and Gertler, S. (1988) Chemical colitis due to endoscope cleaning solutions: a mimic of pseudo-membranous colitis. *Gastroenterology*, **95**, 1403–1408

McNally, P. R., Maydonovitch, C. L. and Wong, R. K. H. (1988) The effectiveness of simethicone in improving visibility during colonoscopy: a double-blind randomized study. *Gastrointestinal Endoscopy*, **34**, 255–258

Vilien, M. and Rytkonen, M. (1990) Golytely preparation for colonoscopy: 1.5 liters is enough for outpatients. *Endoscopy*, **22**, 168–170

Foreign bodies

Rocklin, M. S. and Apelgren, K. N. (1989) Colonoscopic extraction of foreign bodies from above the rectum. *American Surgeon*, **55**, 119–123

Monitoring

Dark, D. S., Campbell, D. R. and Wesselius, L. J. (1990) Arterial oxygen desaturation during gastrointestinal endoscopy. *American Journal of Gastroenterology*, **85**, 1317

Gupta, S. C., Gopalswamy, N., Sarkar, A., Suryaprasad, A. G. and Markert, R. J. (1990) Cardiac arrhythmias and electrocardiographic changes during upper and lower gastrointestinal endoscopy. *Military Medicine*, **155**, 9–11

Therapy

anardhana, R., Bowman, D., Brodmerkel, G. J., Jr., Agarwal, R. M., Gregory, D. H. and Ashok, P. S. (1987) Cecal volvulus: decompression and detorsion with a colonoscopically placed drainage tube. *American Journal of Gastroenterology*, **82**, 912–914

Jensen, D. M. and Machicado, G. A. (1988) Diagnosis and treatment of severe hematochezia. The role of urgent colonoscopy after purge. *Gastroenterology*, **95**, 1569–1574

Krasner, N. (1989) Laser therapy in the management of benign and malignant tumours of the colon and rectum. *International Journal of Colorectal Disease*, **4**, 2–5

Mellow, M. H. (1989) Endoscopic laser therapy as an alternative to palliative surgery for adenocarcinoma of the rectum: comparison of costs and complications. *Gastrointestinal Endoscopy*, **35**, 283–287

Nano, D., Prindville, T., Pauly, M., Chow, H. and Trudeau, W. (1987) Colonoscopic therapy of acute pseudo-obstruction of the colon. *American Journal of Gastroenterology*, **82**, 145–148

Electrosurgery

Barlow, D. E. (1982) Endoscopic applications of electrosurgery: a review of the basic principles. *Gastrointestinal Endoscopy*, **28**, 73–76

Polyps

Jass, J. R. (1989) Do all colorectal carcinomas arise in pre-existing adenomas *World Journal of Surgery*, **13**, 45–51

Waye, J. D. (1987) Techniques of polypectomy: hot biopsy forceps and snare polypectomy. *American Journal of Gastroenterology*, **82**, 615–618

Williams, C. B. (1991) Small polyps: the virtue and dangers of hot biopsy *Gastrointestinal Endoscopy*, **37**, 394–395

Complications

Browter, R. A. (1988) BICAP-induced colonic perforation. *Gastrointestinal Endo scopy*, **34**, 58

Habr-Gama, A. and Waye, J. D. (1989) Complications and hazards of gastro intestinal endoscopy. *World Journal of Surgery*, **13**, 193–201

Levine, E. and Wetzel, L. H. (1987) Splenic trauma during colonoscopy. *American Journal of Roentgenology*, **149**, 339–340

Reiersen, O., Skjoto, J., Jacobsen, C. D. and Rosseland, A. R. (1987) Complica tions of fiberoptic gastrointestinal endoscopy: five years' experience in a central hospital. *Endoscopy*, **19**, 1–6

4

Endoscopic retrograde cholangiopancreatography (ERCP)

The evolution of ERCP (the ability to opacify the biliary tree and pancreatic ductal system through the duodenal papilla) has been one of the great achievements of modern endoscopy. Initially, ERCP was a purely diagnostic technique. However, since the first report of endoscopic sphincterotomy (papillotomy) by Kawai in 1974, an amazing variety of therapeutic uses have developed.

ERCP requires unique endoscopic skills. The technique for maneuvering a side-viewing endoscope (duodenoscope) is very different from that used in gastroscopy with an end-viewing instrument. It is not an easy technique to learn; the movements of the endoscope and control knobs are far from intuitive. A finely developed sense of position (spatial awareness) derived from two-dimensional images is one of the basic requirements. There is a long learning curve. Such is the diversity of anatomic variation and pathology in the biliary tree and pancreas that proficiency in diagnostic and basic therapeutic ERCP requires experience of at least one hundred procedures.

The skills required to master diagnostic and therapeutic ERCP cannot be learned from a book. Accordingly, this chapter is intended to provide an overview rather than stepwise instruction. The endoscopist who performs ERCP must have broad training in the management of biliary and pancreatic disorders, and an appreciation of the benefits of close collaboration with colleagues in surgery and interventional radiology.

Indications for ERCP

Diagnostic ERCP is generally indicated in:

1 Evaluation of the jaundiced patient suspected of having biliary obstruction.
2 Evaluation of the patient without jaundice whose clinical presentation suggests pancreatic or biliary tract disease.

3 Evaluation of signs of symptoms suggesting pancreatic malignancy when results of indirect imaging (e.g. ultrasound (US), computerized tomography (CT), magnetic resonance imaging (MRI)) are equivocal or normal.
4 Evaluation of recurrent or persistent pancreatitis of unknown etiology.
5 Preoperative evaluation of the patient with chronic pancreatitis.
6 Evaluation of possible pancreatic pseudocyst undetected by CT or US and for known pseudocyst prior to planned surgical therapy.
7 Evaluation of the sphincter of Oddi by manometry.

Diagnostic ERCP is generally **not** *indicated in:*

1 Evaluation of abdominal pain of obscure origin in the absence of objective findings which suggest biliary tract or pancreatic disease.
2 Evaluation of suspected gallbladder disease without evidence of bile duct disease.
3 As further evaluation of pancreatic malignancy which has been demonstrated by US or CT, unless management will be altered.
[4 Routine evaluation of the biliary tree prior to laparoscopic cholecystectomy, *unless* there is radiologic and/or biochemical evidence of choledocholithiasis. (Added by author; not in current ASGE guidelines.)]

Therapeutic ERCP is generally indicated for:

1 Endoscopic sphincterotomy
    (a) Choledocholithiasis (e.g. postcholecysectomy patients or patients with intact gallbladders who are not candidates for surgery). [Also, as an adjunct to laparoscopic cholecystectomy, either pre- or postoperatively, when stones are present. (Added by author; not in ASGE guidelines.)]
    (b) Papillary stenosis or sphincter of Oddi dysfunction.
    (c) Prior to placement of biliary stent or balloon dilatation of biliary stricture.
    (d) Sump syndrome.
    (e) Choledochocele.
    (f) Ampullary carcinoma in patients who are not candidates for surgery.
    [(g) To provide access for endoscopic choledochoscopy and its therapeutic applications (e.g. laser lithotripsy). (Added by author; not in ASGE guidelines.)]
2 Stent placement across benign or malignant strictures, biliary fistula or in high-risk patients with large, unremovable common duct stones.
3 Balloon dilatation of biliary strictures.
4 Nasobiliary drain placement for prevention or treatment of acute cholangitis or infusion of chemical agents for common duct stone dissolution.

The hardware

Endoscopes

ERCP is performed using a side-viewing endoscope (duodenoscope) (Figure 4.1). The field of view is large in the vertical plane to provide a generous view of the medial wall of the descending (2nd) duodenum (Figure 4.2). The duodenoscope has a special modification at the lower end of the instrument channel, an elevator that moves up and down (Figure 4.3). This provides a means of adjusting the angle of 'attack' of cannulae

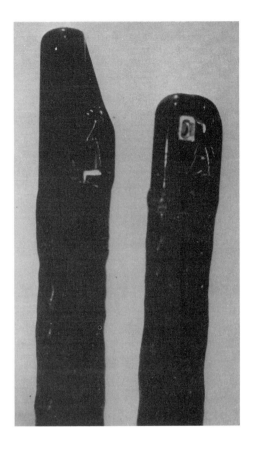

Figure 4.1 Side-viewing endoscope (duodenoscope)

and other accessories being inserted into the main duodenal papilla. The potential for therapeutic intervention has increased as instrument channels have become larger. The standard channel is about 2.8 mm in diameter. For placement of endoprostheses of 10 and 11.5 Fr, a 3.7–4.2 mm channel duodenoscope is required. Even larger stents (e.g. 14 Fr) can be placed using special duodenoscopes with a 5.5 mm diameter instrument channel. However, these are rarely used.

   In patients who have had a Billroth II gastrectomy, ERCP is somtimes performed with a standard end-viewing endoscope, as this may be the only way to visualize the main duodenal papilla at an angle suitable for cannulation. However, it is almost always preferable to use a side-viewing endoscope, even in cases of anatomic difficulty, as the end-viewing instrument lacks an elevator.

Accessories

The standard ERCP cannula is 5 Fr, 200 cm long and has a series of 3 mm etched markings at the tip (Figure 4.4). These markings help the endoscopist to gauge depth of cannulation. The cannula has built-in curvature to aid

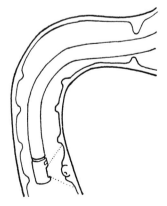

Figure 4.2 The field of view of the duodenoscope

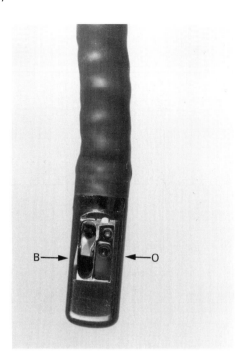

Figure 4.3 Tip of duodenoscope. B, elevator or 'bridge'; O, light source and optics

insertion. A variety of specialized cannula tips are available, including the ball tip and the metal tip (Figure 4.5). The ball tip catheter is said to be the easiest for the novice to use. Taper tip and metal tip catheters have specialized indications; in view of their considerable potential for causing trauma they should be used with great care, especially by inexperienced endoscopists.

The *papillotome* (or sphincterotome) is a cannula specially modified for cutting: a wire at the distal end conveys current to the tissue being cut.

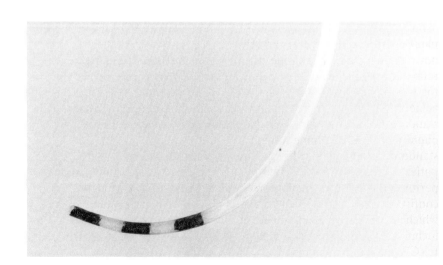

Figure 4.4 Standard ERCP cannula with markings

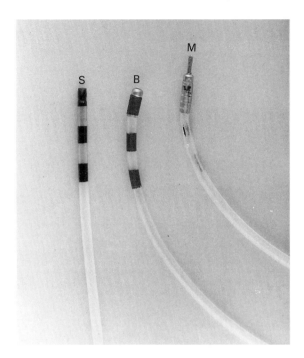

Figure 4.5 ERCP catheters. S, standard; B, ball tip; M, metal tip

Sphincterotomy is used to open up the distal common bile duct (CBD) by creating a vertical cut in the papillary apparatus. Endoscopic papillotomy is the prelude to many therapeutic ERCP procedures. Papillotomes come in a variety of shapes and sizes. Standard papillotomes have 20–30 mm of wire exposed (Figure 4.6). Contrast material will exit through the side-holes in a standard papillotome. This makes a deep cannulation necessary if duodenal spillage of contrast is to be avoided. More recent wire-guided papillotome designs have overcome this problem. A popular variant is the 'long-nosed' papillotome, initially devised for trainees; it ensures deep cannulation of the CBD throughout the procedure (Figure 4.7). Short wire papillotomes (e.g. 10 mm) can be useful in certain circumstances, but are not recommended for routine use. The papillotome wire is tightened and relaxed using the snare-type cannula handle. When the wire is tightened, the papillotome is 'bowed' (Figure 4.8). The upward angulation of the tip achieved by this bowing action is greater than can be achieved with a standard ERCP cannula. For this reason, experienced endoscopists frequently use a papillotome to gain access to the CBD when they fail with a standard cannula. If it is likely that papillotomy will be required, e.g. the patient is known to have CBD stones, the diagnostic cholangiogram can be performed with the papillotome. When the need for papillotomy is confirmed, the cut can then be made without having to change cannulae, which risks losing deep cannulation of the common bile duct. The technique of endoscopic papillotomy is discussed below (Therapeutic ERCP).

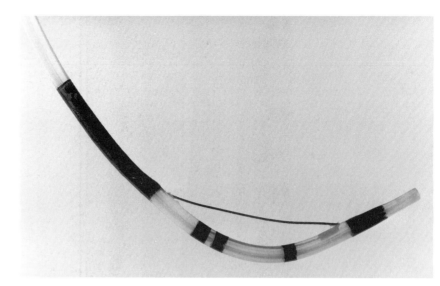

Figure 4.6 Standard papillotome (20 mm wire)

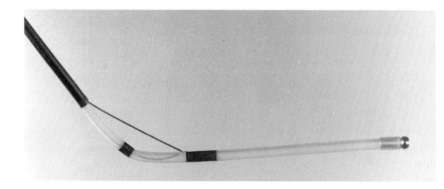

Figure 4.7 Long-nosed papillotome

Guidewires are used increasingly to gain and maintain access to the CBD and pancreatic duct (PD) for both diagnostic and therapeutic procedures. The standard guidewire is 0.035 inches in diameter and up to 400 cm long. As guidewires are inherently floppy, they are usually advanced through plastic catheters (Figure 4.9). Guidewires are essential for endoprosthesis and nasobiliary drain placement. Certain papillotomes can be advanced over a guidewire, which ensures access to the bile duct during and after the cut. Thin guidewires (e.g. 0.025 and 0.018 inches in diameter) are very floppy indeed. Contrary to expectations, they are not ideal for negotiating tight strictures, as thin wires transmit axial forces poorly. However, a thin guidewire can provide access for biliary manometry (i.e. the wire is positioned in the bile duct through a standard catheter, which is then exchanged for the manometry catheter) and dorsal PD cannulation and stenting. The standard 0.035 inch guidewire is usually advanced through a 6 or 7 Fr polyethylene catheter. In stenting parlance, this combination is

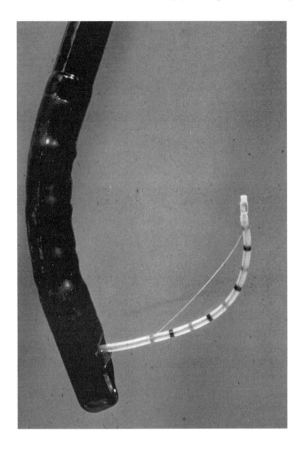

Figure 4.8 Bowed
papillotome

referred to as a 'prewired inner catheter'. Guidewires can cause considerable damage in inexperienced or careless hands. Repeatedly advancing a guidewire against resistance may result in the formation of a false passage, creating problems ranging from submucosal injection of contrast to retroperitoneal perforation. A soft-tipped guidewire, e.g. the so-called J-wire, reduces trauma but may be less effective in negotiating tight strictures. One recent and increasingly popular variant of this is the so-called Glidewire™, which has a slippery surface.

Accessories used to retrieve stones from the biliary tree (and occasionally, the PD) include *occlusion balloons* and *basket catheters*. The

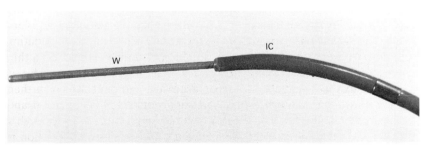

Figure 4.9 0.35 inch wire
(W) through a 7 Fr plastic
inner catheter (IC)

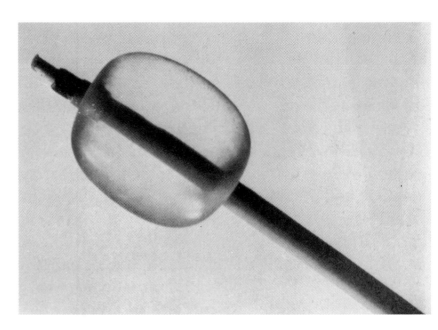

Figure 4.10 Occlusion
balloon

standard occlusion balloon (Figure 4.10) is 12 mm in diameter when fully inflated. Larger (up to 20 mm) and smaller balloons are also available. In addition to their role in extracting stones and debris, occlusion balloons are useful for occlusion cholangiography.

Occlusion cholangiography

When a common hepatic duct or hilar stricture is present, contrast injected through a standard catheter may preferentially fill the gallbladder or simply empty into the duodenum. By inflating an occlusion balloon just below the stricture (Figure 4.11a, b), contrast can be injected through it under pressure. Continued injection of contrast will outline the biliary tree proximal to the stricture. Care should be taken not to fully fill the dilated intrahepatic ducts during occlusion cholangiography, as distending an already obstructed system increases the risk of cholangitis and bacteremia. With the stricture outlined, an inner catheter can be passed over a guidewire into the obstructed system, which is then decompressed. Samples of the bile should be sent for cytology and bacteriologic examination. Further opacification of the proximal biliary tree can then be completed safely by contrast injection through the plastic inner catheter. Occlusion cholangiography is also useful when there is a large papillary orifice (e.g. after previous sphincterotomy) or surgical biliary diversion (e.g. choledochoduodenostomy) (Figure 4.12).

The balloon is inflated just inside the orifice, to prevent leakage of injected contrast. Occlusion balloons are easily damaged. They are effective for removing small stones and debris ('sweeping the duct') after papillotomy, but rarely helpful when a large (> 15 mm) stone needs to be

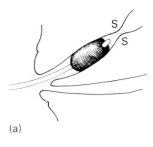

(a)

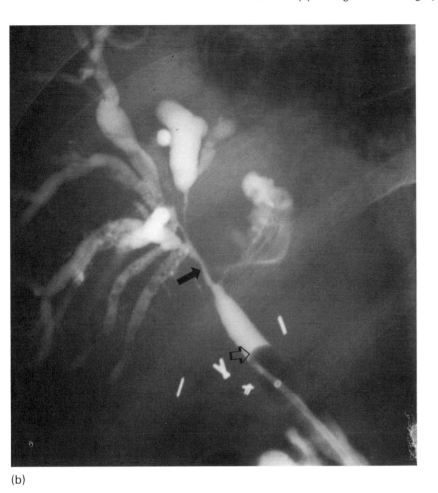

(b)

Figure 4.11 (a) Occlusion cholangiography. The inflated balloon occludes the bile duct just below a stricture (S), allowing contrast to be injected under pressure. (b) Occlusion cholangiogram. Occlusion balloon inflated (open arrow) below tight hilar stricture (closed arrow)

dislodged. The balloon may break when pulled against the stone, or slip past it. To avoid rupturing the balloon by dragging it over an 'up' elevator (Figure 4.13), put the elevator fully 'down' before inserting or withdrawing the tip of the balloon catheter.

Knowing when catheters, etc. are at the end of the duodenoscope. With the elevator in the 'down' position, you cannot see where a catheter is going, or what length has been advanced into the duodenum (Figure 4.14). To avoid this problem, the elevator should be raised as the accessory is advanced down the instrument channel. When the tip of the catheter meets the 'up' elevator, there will be sudden resistance. The elevator should be lowered, the catheter advanced a few centimeters, and the elevator raised again. The catheter will then come into view between the endoscope and the duodenal wall. It is wise to inflate an occlusion balloon in the duodenum to test its patency *before* advancing it into the bile duct (or PD).

Retrieval baskets look like snares, except that they have more wires (3–8) (Figure 4.15). They are designed to capture stones within the wires, which

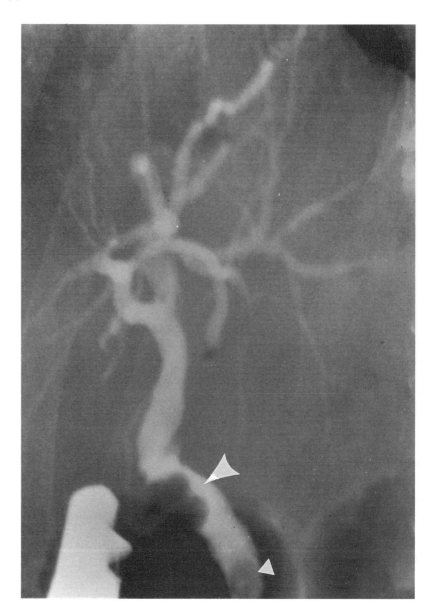

Figure 4.12 Occlusion cholangiogram through a choledochoduodenostomy. Balloon (inflated) is straddling orifice (large arrow). Note filling defect (stone) present in biliary 'sump' (small arrow)

are tightened to form an enclosing basket. The stones can then be extracted into the duodenum. Baskets are useful, but like occlusion balloons, they have certain limitations. Stones of 15 mm diameter or larger are difficult to extract intact from the bile duct after standard papillotomy. Lesser stones may present problems if the papillotomy is too small. It is possible for a basket to become stuck. This can result from being greedy: if you try to remove a whole column of stones, they may end up packed in the distal bile duct, with the basket trapped above (Figure 4.16). Whenever possible, try to remove a column of stones one by one, the most distal first.

You may also get stuck after opening a basket in the bile duct to allow contrast injection (baskets have to be opened a little way before contrast can be injected through them). If a stone is trapped accidentally during this procedure, it may prove impossible to release.

A catheter with multiple channels (multilumen) is used for *manometry*. Using a perfusion system, pressure differences can be detected between the duodenum and the sphincter of Oddi, the CBD and the PD. Manometry is used to identify patients with papillary stenosis or dysfunction who may benefit from endoscopic papillotomy. This type of manometry is technically difficult. As narcotic drugs must be avoided (they affect sphincter of Oddi function) the patient may be less cooperative than usual. A rapid, atraumatic, deep cannulation is needed to avoid trauma to the papilla, which would also affect the result. Some endoscopists perform the initial cannulation with a standard cannula through which a thin guidewire (e.g. 0.018 inches) is passed. The cannula is removed, leaving the guidewire deep in the desired duct. The manometry catheter can then be advanced into position over the guidewire. The technical aspects of biliary, pancreatic and sphincter of Oddi manometry are beyond the scope of this book.

Nasobiliary drains and *endoprostheses* (stents) are described below (Therapeutic ERCP). *Cytology brushes* are available for use during ERCP, the newer types being inserted over a guidewire. Brushing a biliary or pancreatic stricture may yield malignant cells. A cytologic diagnosis of cancer may spare the patient percutaneous biopsy or surgery.

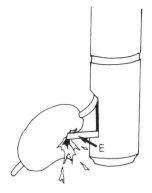

Figure 4.13 A retrieval balloon ruptured over an elevator (E) left in the 'up' position

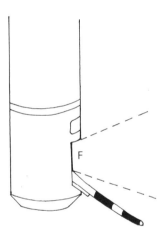

Figure 4.14 Field of view (F) of the duodenoscope renders catheters invisible when the elevator is in the full 'down' position

X-ray facilities

High quality fluoroscopy and radiograms are essential for ERCP. No matter how skilled the endoscopist, poor X-ray facilities will prejudice the successful outcome of diagnostic and (especially) therapeutic ERCP. Anyone who has suffered the frustration of being unable to see catheters and guidewires because of poor fluoroscopy will appreciate the need to use the best equipment available. Endoscopy units with a high volume of

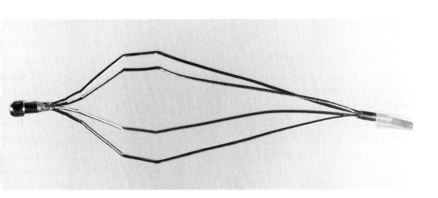

Figure 4.15 Basket catheter

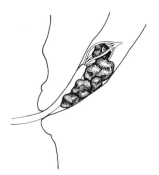

Figure 4.16 Retrieval basket containing a stone trapped above a column of bile duct stones

ERCP cases can justify the installation of dedicated fluoroscopy equipment, including a film processor. In the ideal situation, endoscopic and fluoroscopic images are displayed side by side on monitors directly in front of the endoscopist.

In all but the largest hospitals and clinics, endoscopists and their assistants perform ERCP in the X-ray department, where the assistance of an interested radiologist, or a skilled X-ray technologist is invaluable. There are certain problems that may arise when performing ERCP in another department. First, you need enough time: avoid pressure to complete the procedure quickly and vacate the room. Be realistic when you estimate the amount of time you require and never promise anyone 'a quick ERCP'. Second, the fluoroscopy monitor should be directly in your view, preferably on the other side of the X-ray table (Figure 4.17). It is an unnecessary burden to look at an X-ray monitor over your shoulder, as can happen if the room is set up for standard GI radiology. Third, make sure that resuscitation equipment of the standard you expect in the endoscopy unit is easily accessible. Finally, as the X-ray department may not have a recovery facility for monitoring patients after endoscopic procedures, alternative arrangements must be made. These could include admission to a short-stay ward or the recovery area of the surgical operating room.

It is not enough for the ERCP endoscopist to be skilled at passing the duodenoscope and cannulating the papilla: he or she must learn to interpret fluoroscopy and radiograms. As most decisions concerning therapeutic intervention at ERCP are made 'on the spot', endoscopists need to recognize radiologic findings. As it is rare to have the assistance of an experienced radiologist during every ERCP, the endoscopist must be self-sufficient. However, this does not imply that the radiologist is redundant: far from it. All ERCP films should be sent for formal radiologic interpretation, otherwise important information may be missed. The radiologist's report must be reviewed by the endoscopist to insure that radiologic findings missed at ERCP are noted and, if necessary, acted upon.

Using contrast media

It is appropriate at this point to mention *contrast media*. Water-soluble agents, such as Conray™, (meglumine iothalamate) are used. To outline small diameter ducts, dense contrast (i.e. 50% or greater) is preferable. However, dense contrast in a dilated duct can obscure filling defects, such as stones, and make it difficult to see guidewires and catheters. For this reason, dilute contrast (e.g. 15–30%) should be used when looking for bile duct stones or performing any therapeutic procedure. Your assistant should prepare a 20 ml syringe of standard contrast and another of dilute contrast for ERCP, so that you can switch between them if necessary. Iodine-containing contrast media are unlikely to cause allergic reactions during ERCP, as very little gets into the bloodstream. However, patients with a history of contrast allergy should receive steroid prophylaxis (e.g. a

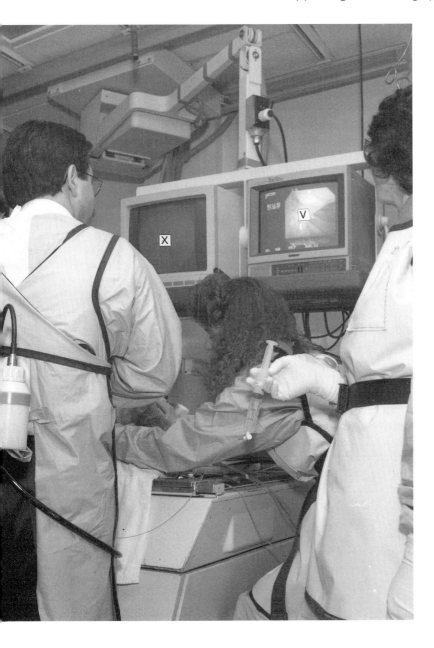

Figure 4.17 Ideal positioning of X-ray (X) and video (V) monitors, directly across from endoscopist

loading' dose of prednisone given in divided doses over 24–36 hours) and an antihistamine agent may be given with the intravenous sedation. There is considerable interest in the use of non-ionic contrast media. It has been suggested that these may reduce the likelihood of post-ERCP pancreatitis. However, as non-ionic contrast media (such as Isovue; iopamidol) are considerably more expensive than standard contrast media their use has been limited.

One of the responsibilities of the endoscopy assistant is to ensure that all air is purged from syringes and catheters prior to contrast injection. Air bubbles appear as radiolucent defects that may be indistinguishable from stones, so it is important to avoid them. If you suspect that air is present in the cannula, flush it through with a few milliliters of contrast before cannulating the papilla.

Producing quality radiograms is an art as well as a science. You can learn a great deal from working with an experienced radiologist or X-ray technologist. In particular, you should learn how to position the patient to obtain the best views. This includes tilting the X-ray table, obtaining oblique and supine views and bringing the patient back for delayed (drainage) films when appropriate.

Endoscopists performing ERCP should understand the principles of radiation protection. They and their assistants should wear radiation dosimeters, and strive to minimize X-ray exposure. As assistants seated at the head end of the fluoroscopy table may be exposed to X-ray scatter, it is a sensible precaution for them to wear a thyroid collar.

Positioning the patient

It is customary to start ERCP with the patient in the left lateral position. The left arm should be positioned behind the patient's back (Figure 4.18). For those who find this uncomfortable, especially the elderly and obese, a semiprone position is the usual compromise. As the endoscope is advanced into the duodenum, the patient is turned on to the abdomen (prone). The prone position provides a better fluoroscopic view than a semiprone or lateral one.

ERCP anatomy: getting to and identifying the papilla

Contrary to expectations, it is easier to pass a duodenoscope than a standard end-viewing gastroscope, as the former has a smooth, rounded tip. It is acceptable to pass the duodenoscope 'blind', although with experience landmarks in the hypopharynx are easily recognized. The

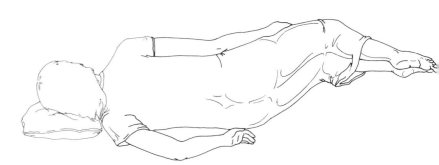

Figure 4.18 Left lateral position with hand behind back

uodenoscope provides a poor view of the esophagus, unless it is patholo-cally dilated. Esophageal pathology is more accurately evaluated using nd-viewing or oblique-viewing instruments. As the stomach is entered, ae endoscopic view is of the lesser curvature in the cardia. By angling the p back and insufflating, a better view is achieved. With experience, the uodenoscope can be advanced through the stomach with minimal insuffla-on, which is more comfortable for the patient. However, if upper GI ndoscopy has not previously been performed, the stomach should be xamined at some point during the procedure. The natural tendency of the ndoscope is to follow the greater curvature. The endoscopist sees the sser curvature, with the angulus (incisura angularis) being a prominent undmark (Figure 4.19). Try to keep the pylorus in view in the 6 o'clock osition. If you lose sight of it, withdraw the endoscope and realign. imply pushing more and more endoscope into the stomach will not get ou through the pylorus. Negotiating the pylorus requires a certain feel for ae position of the endoscope tip. Advance until the pylorus just disappears om view, then rotate the tip down. Combining this 'down' motion with a ttle pressure will advance the tip into the duodenal bulb.

At this point the patient should be turned to lie prone. This alters the ndoscopic view by a 90° clockwise rotation. The duodenum turns post-riorly from the bulb, then inferiorly as it becomes retroperitoneal. This ouble 'right turn' is the key to advancing the duodenoscope tip into the ostbulbar duodenum. These turns are achieved by a combination of lockwise twist on the endoscope shaft, and full right deflection of the tip Figure 4.20). There may be increasing resistance as you advance into the escending duodenum. This results from looping in the stomach (Figure .21). The endoscope should now be straightened by withdrawing. During ais straightening maneuver, it is wise to 'lock' the lateral control knob in ae full right position, to hold the endoscope tip in position. During ithdrawal, the endoscope may advance down the duodenum (paradoxical aotion). In the final straightened position, there should be approximately 0–70 cm of endoscope between the lips and the duodenal papilla. If the ndoscope tip falls back into the stomach during the straightening ma-euver, or at any other time, it may be necessary to turn the patient back n to the left side as it can be difficult to reintubate the pylorus in the prone osition.

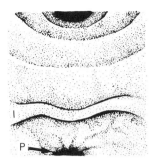

Figure 4.19 View approaching pylorus (P) using a side-viewing endoscope (duodenoscope). The incisura angularis (I) is a prominent landmark

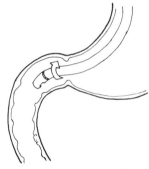

Figure 4.20 To enter the descending duodenum, the duodenoscope should be advanced beyond the pylorus with right angulation and clockwise (right) twist

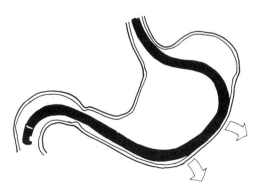

Figure 4.21 Looping in the stomach puts the 'scope in a disadvantageous 'long' position and makes the patient uncomfortable, as there is considerable stretching of the stomach wall

The student of ERCP should learn normal biliary and pancreatic anatomy including variants, which are well described in ERCP atlases and textbooks of radiology. With apologies to Osler, performing ERCP without knowing the relevant anatomy is truly 'to set sail on an uncharted sea'.

Biliary anatomy

Most of us learned in anatomy that the liver could be considered as having four lobes: right, left, quadrate and caudate. However, the arterial, venous and biliary anatomy does not conform to this simplistic external subdivision. A plane called the *portal fissure* passes from the left side of the gallbladder fossa to the left of the inferior vena cava, dividing the liver into right and left; the right has anterior and posterior parts, while the left has medial and lateral. The most recent (and fashionable) anatomical description is the French segmental system, promulgated by the great French liver surgeon, Henri Bismuth. There are eight segments defined primarily by their venous drainge: segment I is the caudate lobe, segments II–IV form the left lobe, and segments V–VIII make up the right (Figure 4.22a). The segmental system has tranformed the practice of hepatobiliary surgery and is fast becoming the standard for describing liver anatomy.

Bile is secreted by hepatocytes into canaliculi and flows through ducts of increasing size to reach the macrosopic biliary system. The serious student of ERCP should be able to identify at least the principal lobar and segmental bile ducts. The right and left lobar (main) hepatic ducts join outside the liver to form the common hepatic duct; this, in turn, becomes the CBD at the level of the cystic duct entry (Figure 4.22b). The gallbladder is a pear-shaped sac (volume about 50 ml) connected to the biliary tree by the thin and often tortuous cystic duct. Gallbladder and cystic duct anatomy is inconstant: endoscopists should be aware of variants such as low cystic duct insertion and aberrant right hepatic drainage directly into the gallbladder. The proximity of the hepatic artery and portal vein to the extrahepatic biliary tree is good reason for caution, and a 'light touch', when guidewires and catheters are being used for therapeutic ERCP. The normal diameter of the CBD is around 6–8 mm. A small increase in diameter is accepted as normal after cholecystectomy. However, a CBD diameter over 10–12 mm is usually pathological, except in the elderly who often have dilated (and tortuous) ducts without evidence of obstruction. Bile release into the duodenum is not continuous but is metered through activity of the sphincter of Oddi, a ring of smooth muscle. There is also a less well-developed pancreatic duct sphincter. The CBD and main PD usually share a final common channel, the ampulla of Vater. However, occasionally two discrete orifices are visible in the main duodenal papilla. Periampullary diverticula, congenital anomalies (e.g. choledochocele, choledochal cyst) and tumors can distort papillary anatomy.

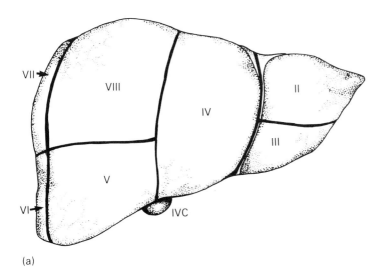

(a)

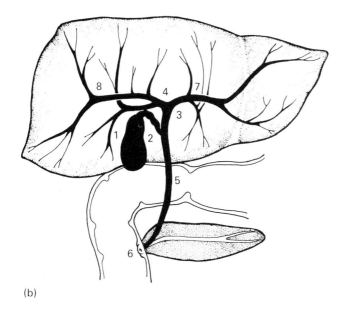

(b)

Figure 4.22 (a) Segmental biliary anatomy (after Bismuth). Segment I not visible on this projection. IVC, inferior vena cava. (b) Biliary anatomy. 1, gallbladder; 2, cystic duct; 3, common hepatic duct; 4, bifurcation (hilum); 5, common bile duct; 6, duodenal papilla; 7, left intrahepatic system; 8, right intrahepatic system

Pancreatic development and anatomy

During embryologic development, the pancreas derives from two buds extending from the primitive foregut (Figure 4.23). These buds fuse to form what becomes the pancreas. Normally, their ductal systems fuse so that the duct of Wirsung becomes the main PD, and the duct of Santorini the accessory one. However, in about 7–8% of normal individuals this fusion is incomplete, which results in the dorsal segment having the dominant system. In this anomaly, called *pancreas divisum*, the majority of

Figure 4.23 Development of the pancreas. (a) The pancreas arises from dorsal (D) and ventral (V) buds off the embryonic foregut. (b) If these buds fail to fuse, the pancreas develops with separate dorsal and ventral duct systems. This is pancreas divisum, which is said to occur in 7–8% of the normal population. The majority of the pancreas drains through the dorsal duct and empties through the accessory papilla. The ventral system is usually quite small. (c) When the pancreatic buds fuse normally, the ductal systems combine so that the majority of the exocrine output is discharged through the main duodenal papilla (at the ampulla of Vater). The accessory duct of Santorini joins the (main) duct of Wirsung near the head of the pancreas

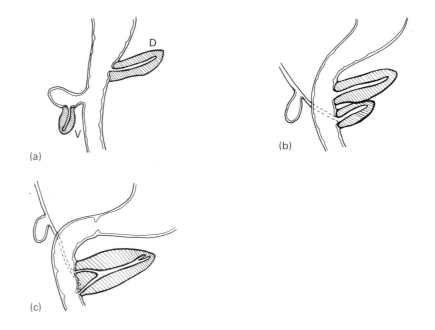

the pancreatic secretion has to drain through the accessory duodenal papilla. Whether or not pancreas divisum is a risk factor for pancreatitis is a hotly debated issue.

The normal main PD (of Wirsung) drains into the ampulla of Vater. The duct starts in the tail of the pancreas, which is designated 'proximal'. It is the distal PD that empties into the ampulla of Vater (Figure 4.24). Endoscopic access to the ampulla of Vater is through the main major duodenal papilla, which is normally located midway down the medial wall of the descending duodenum. There are certain local anatomic features that help you locate the papilla. It is a small, fleshy prominence that lies towards the lower end of a vertical fold. There is usually a transverse fold running across the top of this vertical fold, forming the shape of a 'T' (Figure 4.25). The papilla can be identified by subtle differences in texture

Figure 4.24 Pancreatic secretion flows towards the duodenum. For this reason, the pancreatic tail should be regarded as *proximal* (P) and the duodenal papilla (ampulla) as *distal* (D). Except in the case of pancreas divisum, the majority of the pancreatic secretion flows out through the duct of Wirsung (W), with a small output through the accessory duct of Santorini (S)

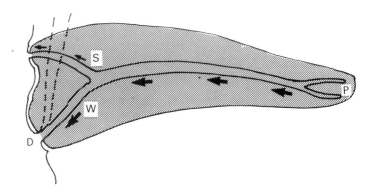

and color compared with the surrounding mucosa. Sometimes it is obscured by an overlying fold which can be pushed out of the way with the tip of a cannula. Careful inspection of the papilla will usually reveal an orifice. Sometimes, two orifices are visible, one above the other: this makes selective cannulation of the CBD and PD much easier. However, these ductal systems normally share a common exit through the ampulla of Vater. From the endoscopist's viewpoint the CBD takes a cephalad course (towards the patient's head) from the ampulla, while the main PD runs almost directly backwards and slightly to the right (Figure 4.26). The appropriate angle is necessary to achieve selective cannulation. The technique required is described below.

Diverticula in the vicinity of the papilla are not uncommon, especially in the elderly (Figure 4.27). If the papilla lies within a diverticulum, access may be difficult or impossible. Once cannulated, the papilla can usually be 'lifted out', making it more prominent and highlighting the course of the distal CBD (Figure 4.28). If a small orifice is visible above the papilla, this may represent the site of a choledochoduodenal fistula (Figure 4.29). These are usually postsurgical, resulting from trauma during CBD exploration. Alternatively, a fistula may result from spontaneous discharge of a CBD stone. If the papilla cannot be identified in the usual position, advance the endoscope into the third part of duodenum, where it may be hiding. Ampullary tumors can greatly distort papillary anatomy. However, although the orifice can often be found at the apex of the lesion, the papilla may also be displaced downwards by mass effect when tumor involves the segment of pancreas above it (Figure 4.30a, b).

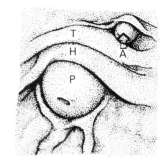

Figure 4.25 Papillary anatomy. P, main papilla; A, accessory papilla; T, transverse fold; H, hooding fold

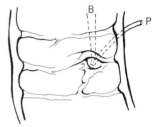

Figure 4.26 Axes of the common bile duct (B) and pancreatic duct (P) from the ERCP endoscopist's viewpoint

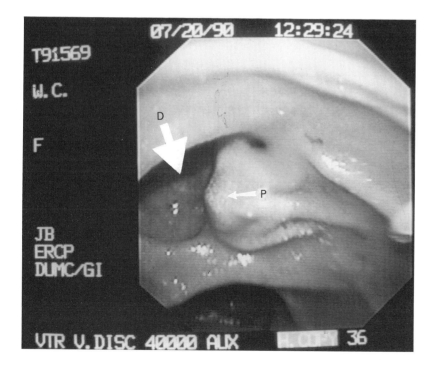

Figure 4.27 Periampullary diverticulum (D). Papilla (P) is identified

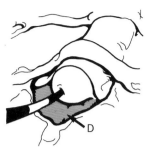

Figure 4.28 Using a cannula to lift the papillary structure out of a periampullary diverticulum (D)

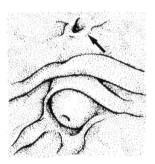

Figure 4.29 Choledochoduodenal fistula (arrowed). This is the usual site of spontaneous fistulation of a bile duct stone, and of traumatic fistula following surgical instrumentation from above (i.e. during common bile duct exploration)

Figure 4.30 (a) Ampullary tumor (T) grossly distorts papillary anatomy. However, the orifice may still be obvious (arrowed). If not, it is often found at the upper pole of the tumor mass. (b) Tumor (T) involving the head of the pancreas adjacent to the duodenal wall may displace the main papilla (arrowed) downwards, making it difficult to locate. A, accessory papilla

The accessory pancreatic duct (of Santorini) empties through the accessory (minor) duodenal papilla. The accessory papilla is small and often difficult to identify. From the endoscopist's viewpoint it is usually located on a fold above and a little to the right of the main papilla (see Figure 4.25). An opening in the minor papilla may not be visible until pancreatic secretion has been stimulated by intravenous injection of the hormone secretin.

Previous gastric surgery can make access to the papilla difficult or impossible. For example, after Billroth II gastrectomy, the papilla can only be reached through the afferent limb of the gastroenterostomy (Figure 4.31), provided that it is not too long. The papilla is approached from below, i.e. the opposite direction to the standard one. Accordingly, it appears 'upside down'. Cannulating the papilla in these circumstances requires skill, experience and not a little luck; papillotomy and stent placement are even more demanding.

I'm at the papilla: what do I do now?

For successful cannulation, you need a nice quiet duodenum to work in. If the patient is moaning, retching and belching, the duodenum will be a sea of motion. Once the endoscope tip is anchored in the descending duodenum, and the patient is lying prone, it is a wise investment of time to stop and 'top up' sedation.

You may also wish to give a drug that inhibits duodenal motility, such as intravenous glucagon, atropine or a hyoscine derivative (unless manometry is planned). Fluoroscopy at this point should show a straight 'scope position (Figure 4.32). If it does not, and there is much more than 70 cm of endoscope down the patient's throat, you are almost certainly in the 'long' position (Figure 4.33). The papilla *can* be cannulated from this position, but it causes the patient considerable discomfort and you lose mechanical advantage. With experience an endoscopist can see and feel this situation developing: the view remains stationary or retreats (paradoxical movement) and there is increasing resistance to forward motion. As in the

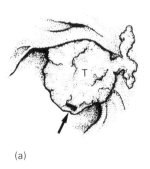

(a)

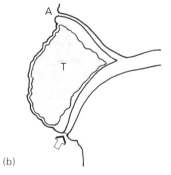

(b)

olon, paradoxical movement suggests looping, in this case in the stomach. If this happens you should gently *withdraw* the endoscope, which straightens out the loop.

When learning ERCP, identifying the main papilla may be surprisingly difficult. Happily, this becomes easier with practice. After straightening the endoscope the papilla may be directly ahead. The transverse (hooding) and vertical folds are identified and the delicate papilla is noted at the bottom end of the 'T'. What if you cannot see any recognizable structure? If you have taken care of motility and patient agitation, the problem may be inadequate insufflation. Until the duodenum is adequately distended, the folds crowd together and fine anatomic detail is obscured. It also helps to 'stand back'. You may be unable to see the wood for the trees: you may be so close to the medial wall of the descending duodenum that you miss the 'big picture'. To distance yourself from the duodenal wall, deflect the endoscope tip 'down' (rotate large wheel up, clockwise). Conversely, 'up' deflection (rotate large wheel down, counterclockwise) brings you closer (Figure 4.34). Remember that in the straightened position the duodenoscope has the right–left wheel locked full 'right'. Releasing the lock will cause the tip to rotate clockwise through an arc from the vertical to the horizontal (Figure 4.35). As this happens, the endoscope will start to slip back towards the proximal duodenum. Once right angulation is lost, the endoscope may suddenly fall back into the stomach as it assumes a completely straightened position. To avoid this, the right–left control wheel should be kept locked during ERCP. Fine adjustments can be made with the lock on. Twist (or torque) is another useful axis of motion (Figure 4.36).

Twist is more easily transmitted to the tip of the endoscope when the insertion tube is straight. This is another reason for ensuring a straightened position before starting ERCP. Twist moves the endoscope tip in a horizontal arc around the papilla. A combination of straightening, fine tuning of the right–left control and a little twist will almost always put you in front of the papillary fold. If, after straightening the duodenoscope, the view is of the descending duodenum as seen from the bulb, you need to advance. The right lock may have to be released before doing this.

What if you are appropriately positioned but *still* cannot identify the papilla? Diverticula can distort the duodenal anatomy. The papilla may lie within or adjacent to a diverticulum. The fold covering the bile duct may be seen running up the back wall of the diverticulum (Figure 4.37). If the papillary opening is in the floor or on the roof of a diverticulum, it may be difficult or impossible to see from the usual cannulating position. The trick is to get close to the papilla by aspirating air to deflate the duodenum; this 'sucks' the endoscope tip into the diverticulum. Once the papilla has been cannulated, it is often possible to make the papillary fold more visible by lifting it out of the diverticulum.

Sometimes the medial wall of the duodenum appears to be a featureless mass of folds. When the usual visual cues are absent, search for the papilla by gently probing the folds with the tip of a cannula. A little patience is often rewarded; the papilla may suddenly appear as you lift up a fold.

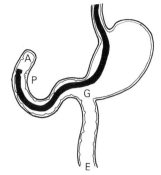

Figure 4.31 ERCP in the patient who has had Billroth II gastrectomy. The duodenoscope must be advanced up the afferent limb of the gastroenterostomy to reach the papilla. A, blind-ending afferent (duodenal) limb; P, papilla; G, gastroenterostomy; E, efferent limb

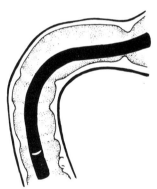

Figure 4.32 Straight 'scope

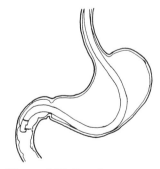

Figure 4.33 Duodenoscope in 'long' position

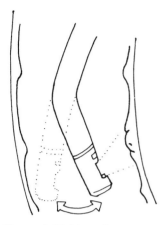

Figure 4.34 Use of up–down control at papilla

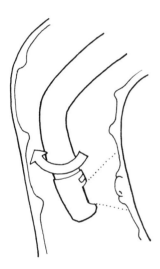

Figure 4.35 Releasing the right lock will allow the tip of the endoscope to rotate from the vertical towards a horizontal position

Selective cannulation

Position is everything when attempting selective cannulation of the CBD and PD. The cephalad course of the CBD requires an acutely angled approach from below, whereas the PD should be approached 'head on' (Figure 4.38). For this reason, the PD is more easily entered than the CBD. Selective cannulation is more than just the triumph of technical skill over papillary anatomy. It is not always necessary or appropriate to opacify both ductal systems. Once you fill one duct with contrast, the other is often hard to cannulate. This may be because the ampullary septum is deflected, closing off the unfilled duct (Figure 4.39). As you would expect, selective cannulation is essential for therapeutic ERCP.

Entering the common bile duct

To enter the CBD, position the endoscope tip *below* the papilla so that the cannula can be inserted in a cephalad orientation (Figure 4.40). If you advance the endoscope too far, the angle will become too acute for cannulation and the papilla may disappear from view. If the position looks and feels all wrong, start again. It can help to partially deflate the duodenum and withdraw the endoscope. Aim to cannulate in the longitudinal axis of the duct, as tangential cannulation rarely succeeds (Figure 4.41). Some fine tuning of lateral tip deflection may be required. The lock should be left on the lateral control wheel. Remember, you are starting with full tip deflection to the right; some of this angulation may have to be removed to get aligned with the CBD. Finding the correct cephalad approach requires skill and experience. Always make small adjustments, or 'mini moves'. An ERCP expert makes multiple small adjustments in each axis to achieve a smooth and seemingly effortless cannulation. There is nothing intuitive about the process; with experience one acquires a feel for it. Until you get to that stage, make one small adjustment at a time; don't try to do everything at once. First, get into a good position below and a little distance away from the papilla, then correct your axis by small adjustments of the lateral control wheel. You can then advance the cannula. Use the elevator: bring the cannula tip up into your field of view by downward rotation of the elevator control wheel. Until you get used to it, the curvature of the cannula is deceptive. *Be gentle!* Don't lunge at the papilla, or repeatedly poke at it in the hope of finding an orifice. The papilla is easily traumatized. The resultant edema and bleeding makes cannulation even more difficult. Inspect the papilla before attempting cannulation. Not infrequently an orifice, or at least a favorable site for gentle probing, can be identified. If you are in the right place, the cannula will slide in easily. You may be rewarded with a deep or 'free' cannulation: a lot of cannula can be advanced with minimal resistance. However, never assume that you have a free cannulation of the CBD. Confirm this by fluoroscopy *before* injecting contrast, as you may be deep in the PD, which is usually undesirable. If you repeatedly enter PD, try using the elevator to

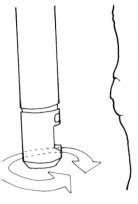

Figure 4.36 Use of twist (torque) around papilla

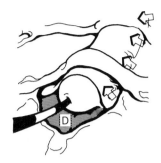

Figure 4.37 Fold overlying common bile duct (arrowed) runs up back wall of periampullary diverticulum (D)

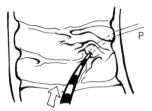

Figure 4.38 Axis for cannulation of pancreatic duct (P)

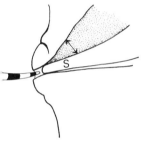

Figure 4.39 When one duct is filled with contrast, the anatomical septum is displaced and may make it more difficult to enter the unfilled duct. Here the bile duct has been opacified (arrowed), causing the septum (S) to press on the pancreatic duct orifice

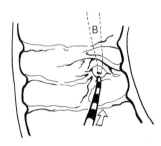

Figure 4.40 Axis for cannulating the common bile duct (B)

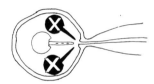

Figure 4.41 Cross-sectional view (from above) of bile duct cannulation: duct should be approached along its axis, and not tangentially ('scopes marked with crosses)

lift the cannula tip just as it enters the ampulla. By forcing the cannula to run along the roof of the ampulla, you increase the likelihood that it will enter the file duct (Figure 4.42).

Sometimes the cephalad angle required for CBD cannulation cannot be obtained with a standard cannula. A standard or wire-guided papillotome can be very useful in this situation. By tightening the papillotome wire, considerable tip deflection can be achieved. However, as the entire length of the papillotome wire has to be out of the endoscope instrument channel, there is more cannula in the duodenum than you may be used to. This can result in poor control of the cannula tip movement. The tip of the

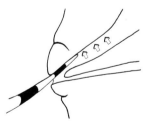

Figure 4.42 Success at biliary cannulation will increase if you aim to run the catheter along the roof of the common bile duct (arrowed)

papillotome can be lifted into the papillary orifice using a combination of tension on the wire and elevator and endoscope tip deflection. Once the papillotome tip is in the papilla, relax tension on the wire a little. This has two purposes: first, it allows more of the tip to advance. If you feel the papillotome advance, relax the wire even more, to allow deep cannulation. Second, as there is often a little 'shelf' in the distal bile duct, an acutely cephalad approach may impact the papillotome tip in the roof of the duct. Relaxing the wire (which reduces the angle of attack) is often enough to let the cannula advance.

The combination of a papillotome and a guidewire may be effective when the papillotome alone fails. Used with caution, a guidewire is a useful tool for gaining access to the CBD. When it does, the papillotome can usually be advanced over it without difficulty. Currently available wire-guided papillotomes are rather stiff compared to standard ones. Some endoscopists may find that the advantages of having a guidewire are outweighed by the disadvantages of a less flexible papillotome. A papillotome, with or without a guidewire, may be used for initial CBD cannulation if you know, or strongly suspect, that papillotomy will be needed. The papillotome allows you to proceed with papillotomy, and the guidewire provides deep access to the CBD. The guidewire can also be used to place a variety of accessories into the bile duct, such as balloons, nasobiliary drains and stents. Contrast can be injected through a papillotome. However, unless you have a deep cannulation, some contrast will inevitably spill into the duodenum through the proximal opening for the papillotome wire (Figure 4.43). *Before injecting any contrast during ERCP, take a control film.* This avoids difficulty in interpreting radiograms, especially if pre-existing calcific densities or contrast materials are present.

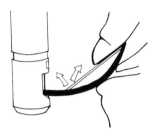

Figure 4.43 Contrast spilling from proximal wire exit hole in papillotome

The cholangiogram

The variants of normal and pathologic findings are beyond the scope of this book. However, there are some basic principles of cholangiography that should be mentioned. First, some diagnostic and most therapeutic ERCP procedures require coverage with intravenous antibiotics. As biliary obstruction predisposes to stasis and sepsis, any patient with obstructive jaundice or cholangitis *must* receive broad spectrum intravenous antibiotics prior to ERCP. These drugs should cover Gram-negative enteric bacteria. One option is to combine a penicillin with an aminoglycoside (e.g. ampicillin and gentamicin). For those allergic to penicillin, vancomycin can be substituted. Some of the new cephalosporins have broad coverage and the added advantage of being less nephrotoxic than gentamicin. The concentration of antibiotics in the blood and liver has been shown to be more important than their presence in bile. The attractive concept of giving the patient antibiotics directly into the biliary tree in ERCP contrast medium has no practical value.

What is a normal biliary tree? The diameter of the CBD and PD increase with age. In the elderly, considerable dilatation of the CBD can be seen without evidence of biliary obstruction. However, in younger individuals, a diameter of 8 mm is regarded as the upper limit of normal. Whether or not the CBD usually dilates after cholecystectomy remains unclear. However, a modest increase in diameter (up to 10 mm or so) is generally accepted as normal in the postcholecystectomy patient. The normal caliber of the common hepatic duct, the right and left main hepatic ducts and the intrahepatic biliary tree become familiar with experience. If present, the gallbladder will fill with contrast provided that the cystic duct is patent. If information about gallstones is required, an erect abdominal X-ray should be performed 1 or 2 hours after ERCP, with the patient still fasting. Similarly, in postcholecystectomy patients delayed films are necessary to assess bile duct emptying in suspected papillary stenosis or dyskinesia. These films should be taken at 5, 15, 30 and 45 minutes following cholangiography. If there is little or no drainage of contrast from the bile duct after 45 minutes, this is defined as significant delay in biliary emptying.

The right and left sides of the intrahepatic biliary tree may not opacify equally. With the patient lying prone, the right intrahepatic system fills preferentially. If additional contrast injection below the hilum fails to visualize the left side, *occlusion cholangiography* may be required (see above, The hardware). A balloon catheter is advanced up the bile duct to just below the hilum. When the balloon is at or proximal to the level of the cystic duct origin, it is partially inflated and contrast is injected under pressure.

Occlusion cholangiography is a useful way to overcome the problem caused by *strictures*. For example, when a hilar stricture is present, it may be impossible to fill the duct(s) beyond it. As the contrast takes the path of least resistance, the gallbladder will fill preferentially. The occlusion technique will almost always visualize a stricture and the ductal system proximal to it (Figure 4.11). Do not force contrast through a stricture into an obstructed biliary tree unless you have some way to provide biliary decompression. If you cannot place a nasobiliary drain or stent, you must have radiologic or surgical back-up. Putting contrast into an obstructed biliary system increases the risk of infection. Whether or not you are able to provide rapid biliary decompression, it is not a good idea to try to fully opacify the dilated system. Forcing a large volume of contrast into an already dilated biliary tree will provoke bacteremia. When possible, attempt to decompress the dilated ducts *before* cholangiography. If a guidewire will pass through the stricture, a 6 or 7 Fr catheter can be advanced over it. This can be used to aspirate bile before injecting contrast.

Trainees frequently ask about *precut papillotomy* as a way to gain access to the bile duct when standard techniques fail. Precutting involves making a 'blind' cut down on to the papilla or upwards from the orifice, as a means of deroofing the intramural CBD (Figure 4.44). It is unfortunate that recent articles in the endoscopic literature have given the impression that this is a safe and straightforward procedure. Being 'blind', precutting is uncontrolled and therefore considerably more dangerous than standard papillotomy. Complications include bleeding, perforation and pancreatitis,

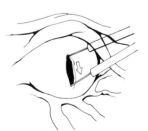

Figure 4.44 Precut (roof of papilla being excised from above)

sometimes with fatal outcome. *Precutting is a potentially dangerous technique that is never justified simply to obtain a diagnostic cholangiogram.* Precut papillotomy for biliary decompression can be life saving in extremely ill patients with cholangitis or pancreatitis due to gallstone impaction. However, it is a technique for experts only! If you cannot obtain a cholangiogram at ERCP, other options are available. These include referring the patient to a more experienced endoscopist, or to an interventional (vascular) radiologist, who can perform a transhepatic percutaneous cholangiogram with external drainage, if required.

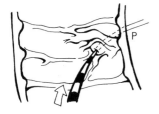

Figure 4.45 Pancreatic duct (P) cannulation

Cannulating the pancreatic duct

Cannulating the PD is usually straightforward. The tip of the duodenoscope is positioned higher (more proximal) in the duodenum for PD access than it is for CBD cannulation. The axis of the pancreatic duct, from the endoscopist's perspective, is directly ahead and slightly to the right (Figure 4.45). Be very careful when injecting contrast: the pancreatic ductal system is easily filled. The aim of pancreatography is to opacify the main PD and its side branches. The latter may be difficult to appreciate during fluoroscopy. It is wise to stop injecting contrast when you see ductal filling out to the tail. Take a radiogram and have it processed. You may find that the side branches have filled; fluoroscopic images often lack the definition to show this. If you continue to inject contrast under pressure, the pancreatic acini are mechanically disrupted with interstitial extravasation of the contrast material. In this process (called *acinarization*) the pancreatic parenchyma 'lights up': the radiogram shows the PD surrounded by indistinct, puffy white clouds. Acinarization should be avoided, as it predisposes to post-ERCP pancreatitis.

What are the causes of failure to obtain a pancreatogram? First, there may be normal anatomic variation. Although entry is regarded as 'directly ahead' for the purpose of cannulation, the PD may take a markedly cephalad course in the head of the gland (Figure 4.46). Some experimentation may be needed to find the best angle for contrast injection. A common cause of a failed pancreatogram is failure to appreciate the presence of a small ventral pancreatic duct. This is easily missed on fluoroscopy. If, despite what feels like an adequate cannulation, contrast spills into the duodenum without obvious PD filling, consider the possibility of pancreas divisum. Take a radiogram during contrast injection: a small ventral PD may be apparent on close inspection. If you suspect the diagnosis, limit contrast injection, as the ventral segment is easily acinarized.

Having identified a small ventral system, the next step is to attempt *cannulation of the accessory duodenal papilla* for access to the dorsal PD. This is technically more difficult than ventral duct cannulation. However, it is not impossible, and your success rate will increase with practice. First, you need to identify the accessory papilla. It lies above and a little to the right of the main papilla from the endoscopist's viewpoint (see Figure 4.25). In pancreas divisum it can be prominent, which may reflect

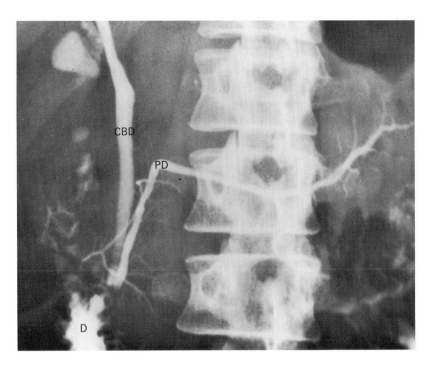

Figure 4.46 Normal ERCP. CBD, common bile duct; PD, pancreatic duct; D, contrast in duodenum

unusually high pressure in the dorsal pancreatic duct. However, the accessory papilla is often hard to find: just an oval prominence on a duodenal fold with no apparent orifice. The accessory papilla may be visible in the 'short position', but it is often necessary to advance the endoscope into a 'long position', which rotates the endoscope tip into a more favorable position for cannulation (Figure 4.47). The tip of the standard ERCP cannula is too thick for accessory cannulation. Suitable alternatives are the metal tip cannula (Figure 4.5) – (not to be confused with a 'needle knife papillotome') and a 5 Fr polyethylene catheter, with or without a 0.018 inch diameter guidewire.

The accessory papilla is easily traumatized by a metal tip cannula. Once there is edema and bleeding, the chances of obtaining an accessory pancreatogram diminish rapidly. The orifice of the accessory papilla is transiently prominent during pancreatic secretion. For this reason it is helpful to give the patient an intravenous bolus of the pancreatic secretogogue, secretin. Within 3 minutes of an intravenous bolus dose, a brief but often profuse outpouring of bicarbonate-rich fluid begins. The accessory papilla becomes more prominent as fluid accumulates in the dorsal PD, then the orifice may 'wink' open. There is a brief 'window of opportunity' to cannulate the accessory PD before the orifice closes again. It can be difficult to fill the duct fully with contrast, which is being injected against a stream of pancreatic juice. Accessory PD cannulation is only indicated if there is evidence of pancreas divisum, when an accessory pancreatogram is necessary to define the anatomy of the dorsal pancreas.

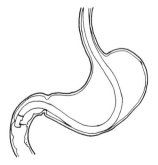

Figure 4.47 Duodenoscope in 'long' position

Local pathology, such as a benign or malignant stricture, may result in failure to obtain a pancreatogram. This may be suspected from the history or from prior imaging with ultrasound or abdominal CT scanning. Pancreatitis can disrupt the main pancreatic duct, causing an abrupt blockage (Figure 4.48). Similarly, intrinsic (ductal) or extrinsic (parenchymal) tumor can have the same effect. When both the PD and CBD are obstructed in the head of the pancreas, malignancy is likely. This radiographic 'double duct sign' results from compression of both ducts as they run close together in the head of the pancreas (Figure 4.49). It is sometimes possible to opacify the PD beyond a stricture by injection of contrast under pressure (occlusion technique) or by advancing a catheter through the stricture using a guidewire.

As discussed previously, over-filling of the PD must be avoided. Under-filling presents its own problems, too. (Contrast drains quickly from the PD, often within 3 minutes, so X-ray films should be taken promptly.) Lesions in the body and tail of the gland may be missed if contrast injection is inadequate to fill the PD. Sufficient contrast should be injected to opacify the side branches of the PD without causing acinarization. Occasionally what appears to be an abrupt blockage of the PD is caused by an air bubble. This may only become apparent on close inspection of the pancreatogram. Pancreatic stones, which are often calcified, and mucus

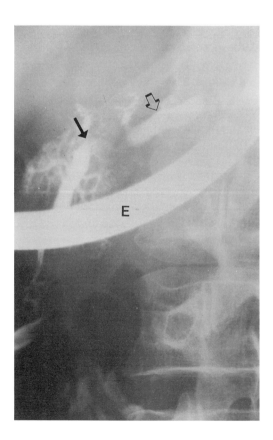

Figure 4.48 Pancreatic duct stricture. Acute narrowing (solid arrow). Dilated pancreatic duct proximal to stricture (open arrow). E, endoscope

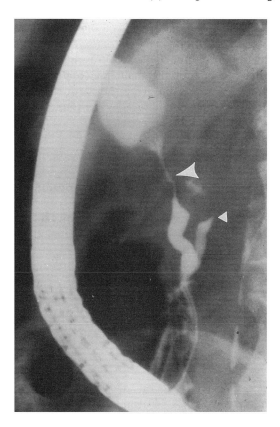

Figure 4.49 'Double duct sign'. Large arrow: tight stricture of proximal common bile duct with gross dilatation above. Small arrow: acutely obstructed pancreatic bile duct

plugs can also cause filling defects. Mucus in the PD is always suspicious for malignancy; if a tumor is not apparent on pancreatography, further imaging, e.g. CT, endoscopic ultrasound, is indicated. Pancreatic calcification seen on a plain radiogram is almost always due to calcified stones in the ductal system.

Retrograde pancreatography in the presence of a known or suspected *pancreatic pseudocyst* requires care and planning: 80% or more of pseudocysts communicate with the pancreatic ductal system. Opacifying a pseudocyst with contrast increases the likelihood that it will become infected. When a pseudocyst is known to be present, it is often helpful to have a 'road map' of the pancreas prior to surgical or percutaneous (radiologic) drainage. Provided that the pseudocyst will be drained within 48 hours, it is acceptable to proceed with ERCP after antibiotic prophylaxis. If a pseudocyst is suspected, make sure that radiologic or surgical drainage will be available should you confirm the diagnosis by ERCP. Successful endoscopic drainage of a pseudocyst through the PD using a nasopancreatic drain (analogous to a nasobiliary drain) has been reported, but this technique has yet to gain widespread acceptance. Endoscopic cyst-gastrostomy and cyst-duodenostomy have been described but are potentially hazardous techniques and are for experts only.

Therapeutic ERCP

A detailed discussion of therapeutic ERCP is beyond the scope of this book. Endoscopic papillotomy, stone retrieval, nasobiliary drain placement and stenting are specialized techniques requiring one-to-one teaching and practice under expert supervision. These procedures will be described briefly.

Endoscopic papillotomy (sphincterotomy)

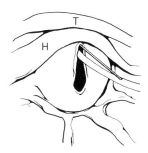

Figure 4.50 Papillotomy in progress. The cut may proceed across the hooding fold (H) but the transverse fold (T) is often the upper limit for a safe papillotomy

This is a technique for opening up the distal CBD, providing access to the biliary tree for a variety of diagnostic and therapeutic maneuvers. A linear cut is made in the longitudinal (12 o'clock) axis of the CBD using a specially modified cannula (papillotome). The papillotome has an exposed wire at the distal end through which electric current is passed. The same electrocautery equipment that is used for colonoscopic polypectomy can be used for papillotomy, with current provided in cutting, coagulating or 'blended' wave-form. As it is vital to ensure correct positioning of the papillotome before making the cut, deep cannulation is required. The length of the papillotomy is also limited by the size of the distal CBD. The aim of papillotomy is to 'deroof' the papilla by cutting through the intramural segment of the CBD.

As a rough guide, if the papillotomy stops at the transverse fold (Figure 4.50), the risk of perforation should be low. However, if the cut strays from the longitudinal axis of the duct, the risk of perforation increases. With the CBD position of the cannula established by fluoroscopy, the wire can be oriented for the cut. Only a very small length of the papillotome wire (less than 5 mm) should be in contact with tissue. This maximizes *current density*, which is inversely proportional to the square of the area of wire (and the cube of the length) touching tissue. A small amount of wire will ensure high current density, with effective cutting and cautery at that site. Coagulation current at a high setting will cut. However, most endoscopists choose to perform papillotomy with blended current. Papillotomy can also be performed with cutting current alone. However, this requires an expert touch as the cut is rapid and bleeding may occur due to lack of tissue coagulation. The papillotomy is made progressively, with a number of short bursts of current. The wire is advanced up the enlarging papillotomy orifice by a combination of bowing (tightening of the wire) and upward movements of the elevator and endoscope tip (Figure 4.51). It is unwise to remove the papillotome from the CBD until the cut is complete, as reinsertion can be difficult or impossible due to local edema. Sometimes the orifice is inadequate for stone removal or other therapeutic manipulation, despite what seems to have been a satisfactory cut. The usual cause is failure to cut the intramural bile duct internally, i.e. the papilla has been deroofed but the bile duct has not been laid open (Figure 4.52). How much internal cutting is required is hard to quantify, and varies from case to case.

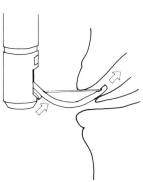

Figure 4.51 Papillotomy. As the cut progresses, the papillotome wire is repositioned by a combination of bowing, use of the endoscope elevator and movement of the catheter itself. 'Up' deflection of the endoscope tip can also be used to advance the papillotome

t is very much a matter of feel. When this internal barrier is breached, here is often a gush of bile, which is a useful signal. Once a papillotomy has been performed, there should be adequate space for catheters, balloons, baskets, etc. to be advanced up the duct. To insert these, aim the ip at the apex of the orifice, where the duct opening lies (Figure 4.53).

Stone retrieval

A major indication for papillotomy is to provide access for bile duct stone removal. The opening has to be large enough to allow the stones to be pulled out intact, unless they are soft enough to crush into pieces. Balloon and basket catheters are used for stone retrieval. A standard occlusion (retrieval) balloon is advanced proximal to the single most distal stone and inflated (Figure 4.54). Dilute contrast should be injected through the catheter at this point to opacify the duct. This makes the stones easier to see. Each stone is pulled out of the duct by steady traction on the balloon catheter. The temptation to pull out an entire column of stones in a single action should be resisted (Figure 4.16), as they may 'bunch up' and block the orifice. Remove a column of stones one at a time. Don't attempt to force a stone through the papillotomy orifice against major resistance. This risks a traumatic extension of the cut, which could cause bleeding or perforation. The balloon is likely to burst if it is pulled hard against a stone. If balloon extraction fails, deflate the balloon and remove the catheter. It may be necessary to extend the papillotomy but a basket catheter should be tried first. This should be advanced beyond the most proximal stone. The basket should be opened just enough to allow contrast injection. If you fully open the basket and unintentionally trap a stone at this point, you may be left in a difficult position. Once you have identified the stones, aim to remove them one at a time, from most distal to most proximal. It is not necessary to fully close the basket over a stone. Indeed, this may work against you if the stone has to be disengaged. Very soft (cholesterol) stones may fragment within the basket. Sometimes this resolves the problem when a large stone is resistant to extraction. Most stones of 15 mm or less can be coaxed through an adequate papillotomy orifice. The likelihood of endoscopic extraction decreases as the stone gets larger. Stones over 20 mm in diameter are a significant problem. The preferred solution is to break the stone into manageable fragments which can then be removed in the standard way.

Mechanical lithotripters are specially strengthened baskets designed to crush large stones. Initial designs were often ineffective but recent developments have been encouraging. Contact fragmentation, using ultrasound and laser energy, and extracorporeal shockwave lithotripsy are promising tools which remain experimental at present.

It is every endoscopist's nightmare to get 'stuck' in the bile duct with a large stone trapped in a basket. The modern solution to this problem is mechanical lithotripsy.

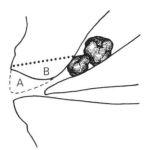

Figure 4.52 If only the external part of the bile duct roof (A) is cut during papillotomy, there may be inadequate space to retrieve stones. An adequate papillotomy requires exposure of the intramural portion of the bile duct (B)

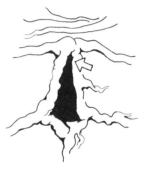

Figure 4.53 Following papillotomy, aim instruments at the apex of the cut (arrowed)

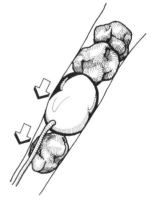

Figure 4.54 The correct way to remove a column of bile duct stones: one at a time, most distal first

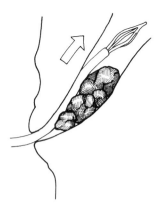

Figure 4.55 To disengage a trapped basket, it should be fully opened and advanced up into the biliary tree beyond the most proximal stone

The trapped basket

If you do find yourself stuck, *don't panic!* Resist the urge to pull harder and harder: this can cause serious damage to the bile duct, including perforation. First, open the basket fully and push the catheter up into the duct. With some back-and-forth agitation, the stone may disengage. When this happens, advance the catheter well up into the bile duct, if possible beyond any stones, before attempting to close the basket (Figure 4.55). Repeat this maneuver several times before abandoning it. However, don't compound the problem by trapping more stones in the basket! If the stones are soft, it may be possible to crush them in the basket. If this does not work, a mechanical lithotripter may. First remove the handle of the basket catheter so that the duodenoscope can be withdrawn over it. A spiral metal oversleeve is then advanced down the catheter until the end is against the stone(s). Using the winding handle of the mechanical lithotripter, the wires of the basket are tightened, pulling the stone against the metal sleeve. This has one of two results: either the stone shatters or the basket breaks. Both resolve the problem of a trapped basket, although if the stone remains intact, biliary drainage remains an issue.

If you do not have the necessary equipment or expertise to perform mechanical lithotripsy, a nasobiliary catheter or stent should be left in place and the patient transferred to a specialist center where the technique is available. It is now rare for any patient with an impacted basket to require surgery for its removal.

Nasobiliary drain placement

Circumstances arise in which adequate biliary drainage cannot be ensured by papillotomy and/or stent placement. For example, stones or debris may be left in the CBD despite papillotomy and attempts at retrieval. In this setting, it is also useful to have a way to perform follow-up cholangiography without subjecting the patient to a further endoscopic procedure. Nasobiliary drain (NBD) placement is the answer. NBDs are polyethylene catheters, usually of 5 – 7 Fr gauge, with a central guidewire, which can be left deep in the bile duct. One type comes with a built-in coil ('pigtail') at the tip which forms when the guidewire is withdrawn (Figure 4.56). The pigtail helps keep the drain within the duct. However it is only useful if the duct is dilated enough to allow the pigtail to form. A second type of NBD is useful in normal caliber ducts. This forms a loop in the duodenum which holds the distal straight segment in the CBD (Figure 4.57). NBD placement is straightforward. The tip of the NBD is advanced deep into the CBD (up towards the hilum) under fluoroscopic guidance. The endoscope is then removed over the drain. This requires teamwork between the endoscopist and the assistant. The assistant slowly withdraws the endoscope by traction on the shaft at the patient's mouth. At the same time, the endoscopist advances the NBD catheter down the instrument channel to prevent the drain being pulled out with the endoscope. The progress of this

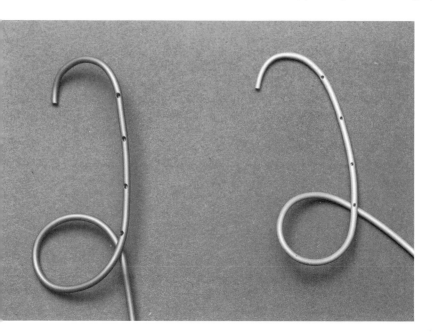

Figure 4.56 Nasobiliary drains

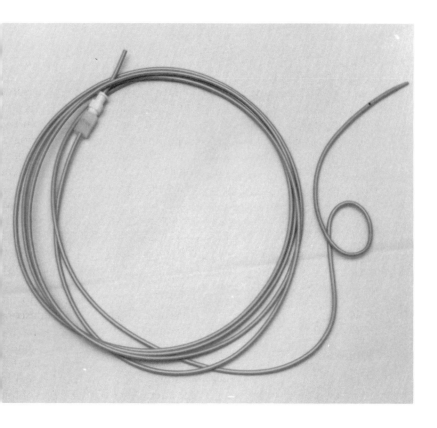

Figure 4.57 Nasobiliary drain with loop that forms in the duodenum

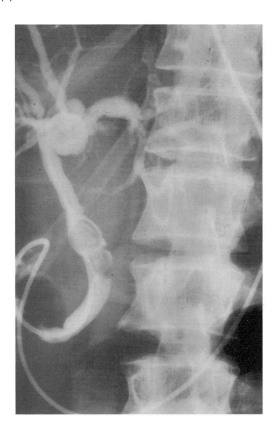

Figure 4.58 Nasobiliary cholangiogram showing drain in place and common bile duct stones

maneuver is monitored by fluoroscopy. At the end of the procedure, the NBD catheter exits the patient's mouth, free of the endoscope. Fluoroscopy should show the tip of the NBD within the duct and a loop of catheter following the greater curvature of the stomach (Figure 4.58). Some endoscopists prefer to leave the NBD guidewire in place during endoscope withdrawal to enhance radiographic visibility. The guidewire should then be removed. The final step is to convert the orobiliary catheter into a nasobiliary one. A standard nasogastric tube (or the custom made tube that comes with NBD kits) is passed through one nostril into the oropharynx, where it is grasped by forceps, or the endoscopist's fingers and brought out through the mouth (Figure 4.59). The tip of the nasogastric tube is cut off with scissors, then the proximal end of the NBD is threaded into it. Once the NBD is deeply seated within the nasogastric tube, the latter is removed through the patient's nostril. When the NBD is freed from the nasogastric tube, nasobiliary drainage is established. There is usually a considerable length of catheter left. Part of this can be coiled and taped to the patient's cheek. The NBD should be strongly secured at the nose by adhesive tape, to prevent accidental dislodgement. The NBD is connected to a collection bag that should be left in a dependent position, to encourage gravity drainage. However, tension on the drain must be avoided.

If little or no bile comes through the NBD, either the tip has fallen back into the duodenum or the connector has been tightened excessively, crimping the tube. It is easy to confirm the position of the NBD by nasobiliary cholangiography. Using a Luer connector, contrast can be injected through the catheter, after first aspirating with a syringe to remove air. If the drain is correctly positioned, you should be rewarded with a cholangiogram. When checking to see if there are stones left in the CBD, use dilute contrast. If there is a large amount of debris in the CBD, e.g. after mechanical lithotripsy, or when a large, soft stone has fragmented during extraction, gentle lavage through the NBD can accelerate duct clearance. Provided that the papillotomy orifice is not obstructed (check this with a cholangiogram), a slow infusion of physiologic (normal) saline through the NBD may wash out persistent debris. Alternatively, the NBD may be flushed periodically. Once the NBD has served its purpose, it is removed by gentle traction.

All endoscopists who perform diagnostic ERCP should have the training and equipment to place an NBD. This simple means of establishing drainage will decompress an obstructed bile duct until definitive treatment can be arranged, whether this is endoscopic (e.g. papillotomy, stenting), radiologic or surgical.

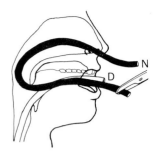

Figure 4.59 Nasobiliary drain placement. After withdrawing the endoscope, the drain (D) is left exiting the patient's mouth. To convert this arrangement to nasobiliary drainage, a modified nasogastric tube (N) is passed through a nostril, grasped in the oropharynx by toothed forceps (or fingers) and pulled out through the mouth. The free end of the drain is then threaded inside this larger tube and both are withdrawn through the nose. In this fashion, the drainage system is converted from orobiliary to nasobiliary

Endoprosthesis (stent) placement

Endoprostheses are plastic (usually polyethylene) tubes inserted into the biliary tree and pancreatic ducts to improve drainage (Figure 4.60). The introduction of large channel ('operating') duodenoscopes in the early 1980s rendered it technically possible to insert large stents under endosco-

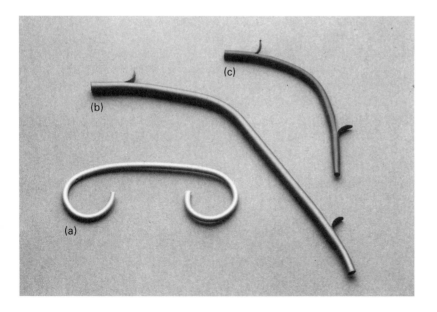

Figure 4.60 Example of polythene stents. (a) 7 Fr double pigtail; (b) 10 Fr straight stent (note curve to fit distal biliary anatomy); (c) 7 Fr straight stent

pic control. Stents have transformed the management of malignant biliary obstruction. They are also useful in the management of a variety of benign biliary and pancreatic disorders. Small stents (7 Fr gauge and smaller) may occlude quickly, often within weeks of placement. This is a function of flow, which varies with the fourth power of stent diameter (Poiseuille's Law). Stent occlusion is associated with the formation of a bacterial biofilm on the lumenal surface. Once a stent clogs, it should be removed and replaced with a new one. Brushing the inside of a clogged stent to sweep it clean is an attractive idea, but it doesn't work. Stents 10 Fr and 11.5 Fr gauge, which are routinely used for biliary decompression, remain patent on average for about 5 months. This is acceptable for patients with pancreatic or other malignancy, whose survival may be considerably shorter. However, using stents to manage benign disease, e.g. large common duct stones, postoperative biliary stricture or benign pancreatic stricture, commits the patient to regular stent changes over many years. These patients should be carefully evaluated, as definitive surgical therapy may be more appropriate.

Stents of up to 7 Fr gauge can be placed using standard 2.8 mm channel duodenoscope; 10 Fr and 11.5 Fr gauge stents require a 3.7–4.2 mm channel; 5.5 mm channel duodenoscopes are available which can take even larger stents (which are rarely used).

Guidewires are the key to stent placement. A standard 0.035 inch guidewire can be positioned deep in the bile duct using a 6 Fr or 7 Fr polyethylene catheter, or through a wire-guided papillotome. Small stents are inserted over the wire alone, using a pusher tube of appropriate diameter (Figure 4.61). The tip of the endoscope is kept close to the papilla, so that the wire and stent are easily visible. The elevator is kept 'up' until the stent abuts against it, then lowered to allow the stent to advance. The natural tendency of the guidewire to advance is counteracted by traction: as the stent advances, the assistant pulls back on the wire. This process must be monitored by fluoroscopy, as the wire has to be kept deep in the duct (beyond the stricture) until the stent reaches the desired position. 'Up' deflection of the elevator after each push helps to advance the stent. The endoscopist must watch for the distal (lower) flap appearing and avoid pushing the entire stent through the papilla, as once inside the bile duct the stent is difficult to retrieve. Small stents almost always advance smoothly through the papilla, and even through tight strictures. Papillotomy is almost never needed for the placement of small stents. When the stent is appropriately positioned, the guidewire is withdrawn. At the same time, the pusher tube is against the end of the stent to prevent it

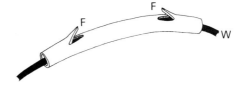

Figure 4.61 A 7 Fr stent over a 0.035 inch guidewire (W). Note proximal and distal stent flaps (F)

being dragged out by friction. Stent placement is now complete, and is usually rewarded with a gratifying gush of bile (Figure 4.62).

Larger stents (10 Fr, 11.5 Fr) are inserted over a 6 Fr or 7 Fr polyethylene inner catheter. In 10% or less of cases a small papillotomy may be required to facilitate stent insertion. A cut of even a few millimeters greatly reduces resistance at the papilla. However, as a complication of papillotomy increases the morbidity of stenting, this should be used only when difficulty is anticipated. A papillotome can be advanced over the guidewire to make the cut. If a wire-guided papillotome is used for the initial cannulation, the process is even simpler. The papillotome is removed and the polyethylene 'inner catheter' advanced over the wire. The tip of the wire and the end of the inner catheter should both be advanced beyond the proximal margin of the stricture (Figure 4.63). A stent of appropriate length is chosen and advanced over the inner catheter–guidewire system. The steps used for the small stent are repeated. However, large stent insertion requires greater physical effort, as the extra layer of plastic (the inner catheter) and the thicker stent increase resistance. The guidewire and the inner catheter must be withdrawn slowly as the stent is advanced. As before, this must be coordinated in such a way that the guidewire and inner

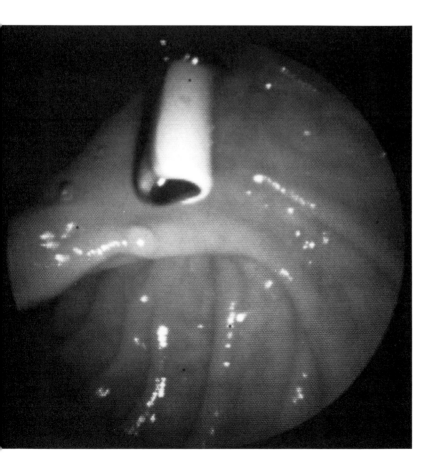

Figure 4.62 Bile draining through a stent

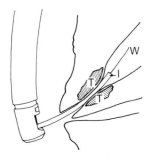

Figure 4.63 The inner catheter (I) with a 0.35 inch wire (W) through it has been advanced beyond the proximal margin of a stricture caused by tumor (T)

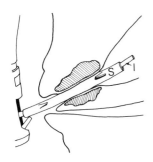

Figure 4.64 The 10 Fr stent has been successfully inserted across a malignant stricture. The 7 Fr inner catheter (I) is left through the stent (S) after the wire is withdrawn and can now be used to aspirate bile and inject contrast

catheter maintain their 'station' beyond the stricture. If they are not withdrawn fast enough, friction pushes them deep into the intrahepatic bile ducts and resistance prevents any further advancement of the stent.

Stent placement requires a team effort between the endoscopist and the assistant. If there is any doubt about whether or not the stent will go through a tight stricture, a dilating catheter can be passed prior to stent insertion. This plastic catheter has the same diameter as the stent: if it negotiates the stricture without major resistance, so will the stent. Once the stent is in the desired position, the guidewire is removed, leaving the inner catheter through the stent (Figure 4.64). This can be used to aspirate bile prior to cholangiography, as it is advisable to decompress the biliary tree before injecting contrast. The bile should be sent for bacteriologic culture and, if indicated, cytologic examination. If further cholangiography is required to opacify the intrahepatic biliary tree fully, this can be done using the inner catheter. Removal of the inner catheter completes stent placement. The position of the stent is then checked radiographically.

Expandable metal stents are currently being evaluated (Figure 4.65). These metal meshes, which expand to about 10 mm diameter (30 Fr), are inserted over a guidewire. The large lumen achieved is an obvious advantage over plastic stents, which tend to clog easily. However, metal stents can occlude due to tumor ingrowth through the interstices of the mesh. Also, precise positioning is critical as, once placed, metal meshes cannot be removed or repositioned.

Endoprosthesis removal

When stents clog, or have served their purpose, they should be removed. This is a simple procedure that all endoscopists should be able to perform. The likely cause of cholangitis in a patient with a stent is occlusion of the endoprosthesis. Intravenous broad spectrum antibiotics should be given. However, sepsis will persist until the blocked stent is removed and adequate biliary drainage restored, either by further endoscopic stent insertion or by radiologic or surgical means. If the distal end of the stent is visible in the duodenum, it should be grasped using a basket catheter (Figure 4.66). This provides better grip than a snare or forceps. Slow, steady traction is then applied. The tip of the stent is pulled close to the endoscope, and both are withdrawn as a single unit (Figure 4.67). This is normally an uncomplicated maneuver. Avoid pulling the stent out rapidly, as the trailing proximal stent flap can traumatize the papilla (bleeding makes it difficult to relocate the biliary orifice). Occasionally, after removal from the bile duct, the proximal flap of a stent will catch on the lip of the pylorus, causing resistance. The stent can be dislodged by pushing the basket catheter back into the duodenum. A stent flap may also catch at the gastroesophageal junction. If esophageal varices are present, it is a wise precaution to withdraw the stent through an overtube, as a stent flap may tear a varix.

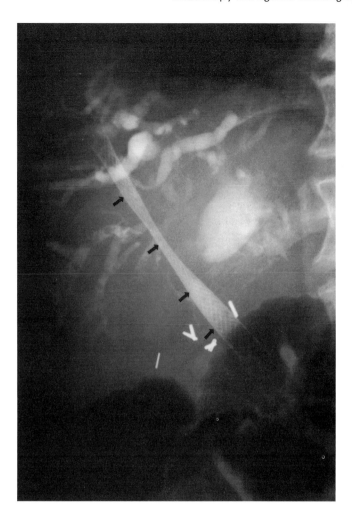

Figure 4.65 Expandable metal stent across hilar stricture (arrowed)

Occasionally a stent will resist basket extraction. Stents may be anchored by fibrous reaction, especially ones that have been present for many months. To increase mechanical advantage, the basket should be advanced as far up the stent as possible. If the basket can be slipped over the stent well into the bile duct, so much the better. The endoscope should be advanced beyond the papilla to align with the axis of the bile duct (Figure 4.68). This will maximize the effect of traction on the stent. When the stent is dislodged, the basket should be opened a little and withdrawn to grasp the stent near the tip. The procedure is then completed in the standard fashion. Replacing the stent is usually straightforward, as there should be ample room for guidewire, catheter and new stent insertion. To avoid the problems of stent occlusion, some endoscopy units offer periodic stent changes at approximately 3 month intervals.

There is a great deal more to know about stenting than can be covered in this brief introduction. The serious student of therapuetic ERCP will find

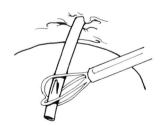

Figure 4.66 Removal of a stent. The distal end of the stent is grasped with a basket catheter

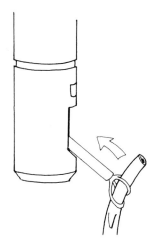

Figure 4.67 The stent, held tightly by the basket, is pulled against the tip of the endoscope prior to withdrawal. This reduces the likelihood of trauma caused by a trailing stent

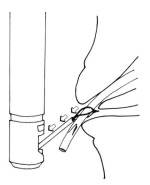

Figure 4.68 For maximum mechanical advantage during stent extraction, the tip of the 'scope is positioned below the papilla, in the axis of the bile duct

more technical detail in one of the large therapeutic endoscopy textbooks. However, it cannot be emphasized too strongly that the only way to learn therapeutic ERCP is by 'hands on' experience under expert supervision.

Complications

No discussion of ERCP would be complete without addressing the complications, which are not insignificant. The morbidity and mortality of diagnostic and therapeutic ERCP are approximately 10% and 0.5–1% respectively. The most common complication of diagnostic ERCP is *pancreatitis*. This means clinical pancreatitis, and not merely hyperamylasemia. The spectrum of post-ERCP pancreatitis ranges from mild (rapidly resolving abdominal pain with or without nausea and vomiting) to life threatening (hemorrhagic pancreatitis). There is no clear understanding of how post-ERCP pancreatitis develops, but recognized associations include repeated cannulation of the PD, acinarization (over-filling) of the parenchyma, biliary manometry and endoscopic sphincterotomy. It is unlikely that post-ERCP pancreatitis can be completely eliminated, as it may occur in the absence of an obvious precipitating cause. Rcently, there has been speculation that hypertonic contrast media may cause or contribute to post-ERCP pancreatitis. However, there are insufficient data at present to support the routine use of non-ionic contrast media.

Cholangitis is a significant risk of ERCP in the presence of biliary obstruction. ERCP performed in patients with biliary sepsis should be covered with broad spectrum intravenous antibiotics given at least 1 hour *prior to* the procedure. A large volume of contrast should not be injected under pressure into an obstructed biliary system. Dilated ducts should be decompressed before attempting to obtain a full cholangiogram. It is essential to establish some form of biliary drainage after injecting contrast into an obstructed system. If a nasobiliary drain or stent cannot be placed at the time, the patient should be kept on parenteral antibiotics. Percutaneous (transhepatic) or surgical drainage of the obstructed system should be performed within 48 hours, where possible. If pancreatography is to be performed to evaluate a pseudocyst, ductal trauma or pancreatic ascites, surgical or radiologic drainage should be readily available. When cholangitis, pancreatic abscess or septicemia following ERCP is found to be due to an unusual organism, e.g. *Pseudomonas*, *Serratia*, endoscope contamination should be suspected. Periodic culture of the duodenoscope air/water and suction channels should identify contamination before it causes a potentially fatal problem. Rigorous cleaning and sterilizing routines for endoscopes and accessories (such as water bottles) should destroy all pathogens, including the viruses of hepatitis B and AIDS.

Bile aspirated from an obstructed biliary tree should be sent to the microbiologist for culture. This can yield useful information about biliary pathogens, including antibiotic sensitivity and resistance.

Hemorrhage and perforation are usually complications of endoscopic papillotomy. However, they can also follow traumatic use of guidewires and other accessories in the biliary tree. Bleeding from a papillotomy site may be arterial or venous. Arterial bleeding is (fortunately) less common than venous. If the papillotome is still in the duct, a brief burst of coagulating current at a low setting may cauterize the offending vessel. As the duodenum fills rapidly with blood there is usually insufficient time to set up a heater probe or inject epinephrine. Fortunately the majority of arterial bleeding settles without radiologic or surgical intervention. When bleeding persists, arteriography will identify an actively bleeding vessel, which may then be embolized. However, this is not always successful, possibly due to the rich collateral blood supply of the duodenum. Sometimes surgery is required to stop bleeding. Factors predisposing to, or exacerbating, bleeding after papillotomy include previous sphincterotomy, papillary tumor, severe coagulopathy and, possibly, portal hypertension.

Although it makes sense to correct known coagulopathy and reverse therapeutic anticoagulation before papillotomy, there is considerable debate about the need to routinely check coagulation indices prior to papillotomy in otherwise normal individuals. Technique is important: a rapid cut with little or no coagulation is more likely to bleed than a slow, controlled cut using blended or pure coagulating current. A rapid, uncontrolled cut (sometimes called a 'zipper') is dangerous and should be avoided. Venous bleeding from the papilla almost always stops spontaneously, although oozing may persist for several days. Injecting epinephrine at the apex of the papillotomy site is technically simple and may slow or stop bleeding. Conservative management, with transfusion if required, is usually successful.

Hemobilia (bleeding from the bile duct) is rare and usually spontaneous. It may indicate liver pathology, such as hepatoma, or follow surgery or liver trauma. Occasionally, hemobilia is noted during ERCP. Friable hilar tumors can bleed after instrumentation. It is possible to cause a fistula between the portal venous system and the bile duct (biliary–venous fistula) by traumatic use of a guidewire. In profuse hemobilia, blood clot may fill the biliary tree, but this rarely causes obstruction to bile flow.

Perforation is a feared complication of any endoscopic procedure. The greatest risk of perforation at ERCP occurs during papillotomy. Perforation can result from too large a papillotomy (often the result of rapid, uncontrolled cut) or from those that stray from the longitudinal (12 o'clock) axis of the bile duct. Trauma from the tip of a guidewire can also cause perforation. Perforation may be 'free' (into the peritoneal cavity) or, more commonly, retroperitoneal (Figure 4.69). A free perforation is usually obvious, as the duodenum suddenly deflates due to decompression into the abdominal cavity. If there is any doubt about the diagnosis, an erect or decubitus lateral radiogram will confirm the presence of free peritoneal air. The procedure should be discontinued immediately and a surgical consultation obtained. The patient should be kept nil by mouth, given intravenous fluid and antibiotics, and nasogastric suction instituted. Laparotomy is almost always indicated following free perforation.

Evidence of retroperitoneal perforation may be missed at the time of the procedure. Odd gas shadows and an indistinct pool of contrast seen on

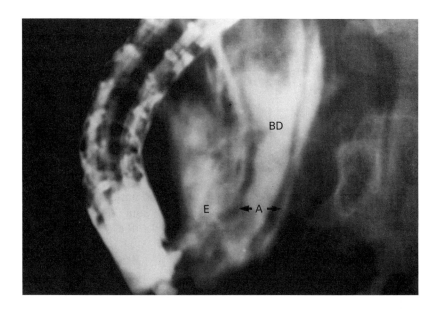

Figure 4.69 Retroduodenal perforation after endoscopic sphincterotomy. A, air outside the bile duct wall (free air); E, retroduodenal extravasation of contrast; BD, common bile duct containing contrast

fluoroscopy should alert the endoscopist, but a small retroperitoneal perforation may not be immediately obvious. It can take several days for the patient to develop abdominal pain, fever, or an elevated white cell count. Surgical drainage is required if retroperitoneal contamination is extensive, although the endoscopic literature suggests that two-thirds of retroperitoneal perforations can be managed medically. Untreated retroperitoneal sepsis has serious consequences, including abscess and fistula formation, so early drainage is appropriate. As therapeutic ERCP patients are often unfit for surgery, their fluid collections and abscesses may be drained percutaneously under ultrasound or CT guidance. Ideally, retroperitoneal perforation should be managed jointly by the gastroenterologist and a sympathetic surgeon.

Submucosal and periductal injections of contrast constitute a limited form of perforation that can almost always be managed medically. They may not be obvious at the time of ERCP. In the absence of post-ERCP pancreatitis, pain precipitated by eating, and fever without an obvious cause are suspicious for localized perforation.

The 'zipper' and how to avoid it

This avoidable complication of papillotomy merits a section to itself. A rapid, uncontrolled cut (the 'zipper') predisposes to bleeding and perforation. It is usually caused by ignorance of how a papillotome works. An inexperienced papillotomist may start a cut with too much wire inside the papilla. As a lot of wire is in contact with tissue, local current density is low and neither cutting nor coagulation will occur. Nothing appears to happen when current is applied, so the endoscopist increases the current. When this produces little or no response, the operator decides that not enough wire is in contact with tissue, and increases the bowing of the papillotome. This pushes the papillotome out of the duct, shortening the amount of wire in contact with tissue and causing a rapid increase in current density. The result is an unexpectedly rapid cut, which is usually longer than desired. There is insufficient time for adequate tissue coagulation to occur, which predisposes to bleeding, and if the cut is long enough, or in an inappropriate direction, perforation may occur.

If nothing appears to happen when current is applied at the start of papillotomy, check the electrocautery circuit. If this is complete, the problem is likely to be too much papillotome wire in contact with tissue. Stop applying current and withdraw the papillotome until only 2–4 mm of wire is inside the papilla (Figure 4.70). If the equipment is working normally, it should not be necessary to increase the power settings. However, if a lot of coagulating current is applied without cutting, the tissue will desiccate (dry out), which makes cutting much more difficult.

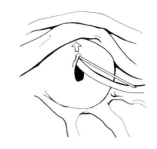

Figure 4.70 Withdraw papillotome until only 2–4 mm of wire is in contact with the roof of the papilla

ERCP after gastric surgery

ERCP is more difficult, and more interesting, after surgical rearrangement of the gastroduodenal anatomy. Ulcer operations may alter the route to the papilla. In particular, the Billroth II procedure and gastroenterostomy for pyloric stenosis mandate a retrograde approach to the duodenal papilla along the afferent limb of a gastroenteric anastomosis (Figure 4.31). Getting to the papilla alone can be quite a feat, especially if the surgeon has left a long afferent loop of bowel. The papilla is approached from below, and thus appears 'upside down' to the endoscopist. It is sometimes easier to cannulate the CBD using an end-viewing instrument than a duodenoscope. Specially designed Billroth II papillotomes may be helpful cannulating the CBD from below, but their positioning is rarely ideal. Fluoroscopy during endoscopy insertion can help identify which limb of the anastomosis has been entered. This is often difficult to determine otherwise, especially if bile is absent due to biliary obstruction.

ERCP after bile duct surgery

One form of surgical bypass for distal bile duct obstruction involves anastomosing the CBD to the duodenal bulb, a choledochoduodenostomy. This opening is initially large but over time it may narrow down to a pin-hole. The bypassed distal CBD can accumulate stones and debris and become a reservoir for infection; recurrent cholangitis in patients with a choledochoduodenostomy may be due to this 'sump syndrome'. The choledochoduodenostomy orifice can usually be identified by advancing the duodenoscope into the 'long position', which provides a better view of the proximal duodenum. If the orifice remains widely patent, an occlusion balloon may be needed to obtain a cholangiogram. If sump debris is present, a standard papillotomy (provided that the distal duct is accessible) and stone clearance should solve the problem.

Increasingly, endoscopic papillotomy is being used to remove CBD stones left at the time of cholecystectomy. In centers with appropriate endoscopic facilities and expertise, this has largely replaced percutaneous basket extraction of CBD stones through the T-tube track (the so-called Burhenne procedure). As the risks of papillotomy are increased when the CBD is not dilated, small stones may be removed without cutting the sphincter. Prior dilatation may be needed to allow access for balloon catheters or baskets. As endoscopic bile duct stone removal, with or without papillotomy, can produce considerable edema of the papilla, the T-tube should *not* be removed immediately after the procedure. Instead, the T-tube should be left on free drainage overnight to allow papillary edema to settle. The patient should then tolerate 24 hours with the tube clamped off (i.e. without pain or evidence of mechanical biliary obstruction) before adequate drainage is assumed and the tube removed.

Nasobiliary drains and stents are frequently effective in sealing off biliary fistulas: e.g. after a T-tube is dislodged or pulled out too soon after surgery, or biliary anastomoses break down. Endoscopic stenting has proved especially useful in managing anastomotic leaks in liver transplant patients. For a normal caliber bile duct, a 7 Fr gauge stent is usually adequate.

ERCP and laparoscopic cholecystectomy

The new surgical technique of laparoscopic cholecystectomy is producing a considerable case load for ERCP-trained endoscopists. Surgeons are requesting prelaparoscopic cholecystectomy cholangiograms and, when indicated, endoscopic clearance of bile duct stones. Routine preoperative ERCP probably cannot be justified. Criteria are available by which patients at high risk of having CBD stones can be identified. Low-risk patients should proceed with laparoscopic cholecystectomy without prior cholangiography. If operative cholangiography reveals a CBD stone, the patient can have ERCP for stone removal the day after surgery. If the bile duct is not dilated, an attempt should be made to remove stones without papillotomy. If necessary, the papilla can be stretched using 'step' dilators or a dilating balloon. Papillotomy in the presence of a non-dilated CBD requires great care and is associated with significantly increased risk of complications (especially pancreatitis). Endoscopic papillotomy with or without biliary stenting has become a useful way to manage biliary leaks following laparoscopic cholecystectomy. Unfortunately, ERCP can diagnose but not treat CBD occlusion by misplaced surgical clips. The use of ERCP in relation to laparoscopic cholecystectomy is still evolving.

Bibliography

General

ASGE Publications, available from ASGE, Thirteen Elm Street, Manchester, MA 01944:

> *Endoscopic Therapy of Biliary Tract and Pancreatic Diseases* (printed August 1989)
> *The Role of Endoscopy in Diseases of Biliary Tract and Pancreas* (printed January 1988)

Cotton, P. B. (1984) Endoscopic management of common bile duct stones (apples and oranges). *Gut*, **25**, 587–597

Cotton, P. B. (1988) Problems in ERCP interpretation. In *Diagnostic Radiology* (eds A. R. Margulis and C. A. Gooding), Radiology Research and Education Foundation, UCSF

Dowsett, J. F., Vaira, D., Hatfield, A. R. W. *et al.* (1989) Endoscopic biliary therapy using the combined percutaneous and endoscopic technique. *Gastroenterology*, **96**, 1180–1186

Fink, A. S., Valle, P. de A., Chapman, M. and Cotton, P. B. (1987) Radiologic pitfalls in endoscopic retrograde pancreatography. *Pancreas*, **1**, 180

Huibregtse, K. (1988) *Endoscopic Biliary and Pancreatic Drainage*, George Theime, Stuttgart

Kawai, A., Akasaki, Y., Murakawi, K., Toda, M., Kohli, Y. and Nakajuma, M. (1974) Endoscopic sphincterotomy of the ampulla of Vater. *Gastrointestinal Endoscopy*, **20**, 148–151

Liguory, C. and Vitale, G. C. (1990) Biliary perestroika. *American Journal of Surgery*, **160**, 237–238

Vaira, D., D'Anna, L., Ainley, C. *et al.* (1989) Endoscopic sphincterotomy in 1000 consecutive patients. *Lancet*, **ii**, 431–433

Biliary strictures

Cotton, P. B. (1990) Management of malignant bile duct obstruction. *Journal of Gastroenterology and Hepatology*, **5**, 63–77

Cremer, M., Deviere, J., Sugai, B. and Baize, M. (1990) Expandable biliary metal stents for malignancies: endoscopic insertion and diathermic cleaning for tumor ingrowth. *Gastrointestinal Endoscopy*, **36**, 55–57

Domschke, W. and Foerster, E. (1990) Endoscopic implantation of large bore self-expanding biliary mesh stent. *Gastrointestinal Endoscopy*, **36**, 55–57

Geenen, D. J., Geenen, J. E., Hogan, W. J. *et al.* (1989) Endoscopic therapy for benign bile duct strictures. *Gastrointestinal Endoscopy*, **35**, 367–371

Hatfield, A. R. W. (1990) Palliation of malignant obstructive jaundice: surgery or stent? *Gut*, **31**, 1339–1340

Pitt, H. A., Kaufman, S. L., Coleman, J., White, R. I. and Cameron, J. L. (1989) Benign post-operative strictures: operate or dilate? *Annals of Surgery*, **210**, 417–427

Stones and cholangitis

Cotton, P. B., Forbes, A., Leung, J. W. C. and Dineen, L. (1987) Endoscopic stenting for long-term treatment of large bile duct stones: a 2–5 year follow-up. *Gastrointestinal Endoscopy*, **33**, 401–412

Kozarek, R. A. (1989) Romancing the stones (editorial). *Gastrointestinal Endoscopy*, **35**, 127–128

Leung, J. W. C., Chung, S. C. S., Sung, J. J. Y., Banez, V. P. and Li, A. K. C (1989) Urgent endoscopic drainage for acute suppurative cholangitis. *Lancet*, **ii** 1307–1309

Martin, D. F., McGregor, J. C., Lambert, M. E. and Tweedle, D. E. F. (1987 Stone extraction after endoscopic sphincterotomy: an active policy is best. *Gut* **25**, 85

Neoptolemos, J. P. and Carr-Locke, D. L. (1989) ERCP in acute cholangitis anc pancreatitis. In *ERCP: Diagnostic and Therapeutic Applications* (ed. I. M Jacobson), Elsevier, Amsterdam

Cytology

Leung, J. W. C., Sung, J. Y., Chung, S. C. S. and Chan, K. M. (1989) Endoscopic scraping biopsy of malignant biliary strictures. *Gastrointestinal Endoscopy*, **35** 65–66

Ryan, M. E. (1991) Cytologic brushings of ductal lesions during ERCP. *Gastro intestinal Endoscopy*, **37**, 139–142

Bile leaks

Cotton, P. B., Baillie, J., Pappas, T. and Meyers, W. S. (1991) Laparoscopic cholecystectomy and the biliary endoscopist (editorial). *Gastrointestinal Endo scopy*, **37**, 94–97

Hoffman, B. J., Cunningham, J. T. and Marsh, W. H. (1990) Endoscopic management of biliary fistulas with small calibre stents. *American Journal o, Gastroenterology*, **85**, 705–707

Stents and stent blockage

Leung, J. W. C. and Banez, V. P. (1990) Clogging of biliary stents: mechanisms and possible solution. *Digestive Endoscopy*, **2**, 97–104

Leung, J. W. C., Del Favero, G. and Cotton, P. B. (1985) Endoscopic biliary prostheses: a comparison of materials. *Gastrointestinal Endoscopy*, **31**, 93–95

Leung, J. W. C., Ling, T. K. W., Kung, J. L. S. and Vallence Owen, J. (1988) The role of bacteria in the blockage of biliary stents. *Gastrointestinal Endoscopy*, **34** 19–22

Complications

Bell, R. C. W., Stiegmann, G., Goff, J., Perlman, N., Ravelli, M. and Norton, L (1990) Decision for surgical management of perforation following endoscopic sphincterotomy. *Proceedings of the Society for American Gastrointestinal Endo scoping Surgeons*, p. 26

Cotton, P. B. (1989) Pre-cut papillotomy: a risky technique for experts only (editorial). *Gastrointestinal Endoscopy*, **35**, 578–579

Cotton, P. B., Lehman, G., Geenen, G. E. *et al.* (1991) Endoscopic sphincter otomy complications and their management: an attempt at consensus. *Gastro intestinal Endoscopy*, **37**, 383–393

Deviere, J., Motte, S., Dumonceau, J. M., Serruys, E., Thus, J. P. and Cremer, M. (1990) Septicemia after endoscopic retrograde cholangio-pancreatography. *Endoscopy*, **22**, 72–75

Hawes, R. H., Cotton, P. B. and Vallon, A. G. (1990) Follow-up 6–11 years after duodenoscopic sphincterotomy for stones in patients with prior cholecystectomy *Gastroenterology*, **98**, 1008–1012

Martin, D. F. and Tweedle, D. E. F. (1990) Retroperitoneal perforation during ERCP and endoscopic sphincterotomy: causes, clincal features and management. *Endoscopy*, **22**, 174–175

Sherman, S., Ruffolo, T. A., Hawes, R. H. and Lehman, G. A. (1991) Complications of endoscopic sphincterotomy. *Gastroenterology*, **101**, 1068–1075

Index